I0413581

# USING CASEMIX SYSTEM FOR HOSPITAL REIMBURSEMENT IN SOCIAL HEALTH INSURANCE PROGRAMME

COMPARING CASEMIX SYSTEM AND FEE-FOR-SERVICE
AS PROVIDER PAYMENT METHOD

SYED ALJUNID, EKA YOSHIDA SYUKRI

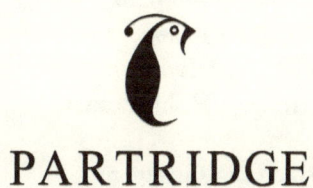

PARTRIDGE

Copyright © 2020 by Syed Aljunid, Eka Yoshida Syukri.

ISBN:        Softcover              978-1-5437-6171-9
             eBook                  978-1-5437-6172-6

All rights reserved. No part of this book may be used or reproduced by
any means, graphic, electronic, or mechanical, including photocopying,
recording, taping or by any information storage retrieval system without
the written permission of the author except in the case of brief quotations
embodied in critical articles and reviews.

Because of the dynamic nature of the Internet, any web addresses or
links contained in this book may have changed since publication and
may no longer be valid. The views expressed in this work are solely those
of the author and do not necessarily reflect the views of the publisher,
and the publisher hereby disclaims any responsibility for them.

Print information available on the last page.

**To order additional copies of this book, contact**
Toll Free +65 3165 7531 (Singapore)
Toll Free +60 3 3099 4412 (Malaysia)
orders.singapore@partridgepublishing.com

www.partridgepublishing.com/singapore

# Contents

# Acknowledgements

In the name of Allah, the Most Gracious, the Most Merciful. Alhamdulillah, Praise to Allah for His Grace and His Mercy in giving me the chance, health, and barokah to complete this book.

This book has been prepared and completed with the valuable contributions of many individuals. We are very grateful for having an exceptional assistance from the support staff and academics in the International Centre for Casemix and Clinical Coding, Faculty of Medicine, National University of Malaysia (ITCC-UKM) and United Nations University-International Institute for Global Health. They have gone beyond their normal duties in helping us to manage data that became the main content of this book. We are grateful to staff of Cipto Mangunkusumo Hospital in Jakarta, Indonesia for their time and tireless efforts to support our work. Special thanks for the staff working in the section that process the hospital payment under Jaminan Kesehatan Indonesia for their support to collect and clean the data for this study.

Dr Eka Yoshida would like to thank and covey her deepest appreciation and great respect to her late parents for all their wonderful love and care over the years; those were the greatest gifts that have ever been given to her. She woud like to express special thanks with deepest love to her lovely family— her husband, Syukri, and her son, Rizqi—for their support and prayers during this study. May Allah SWT bless them with barokah and dignity.

# List of Abbreviations

| | |
|---|---|
| ALOS | Average length of stay |
| Askes | Asuransi Kesehatan = The Health Insurance Company |
| BPS | Badan Pusat Statistik = Central Bureau of Statistics |
| BPJS | Badan Penyelenggara Jaminan Sosial Kesehatan = Public |
| Kesehatan (BPJS) | Health Social Insurance Implementing Body |
| DJSN | Dewan Jaminan Sosial Nasional = National Social Security Council |
| DPR-RI | Dewan Perwakilan Rakyat = The House of Representatives |
| FFS | Fee-for-service |
| KJS | Kartu Jakarta Sehat = Jakarta Health Card |
| IDR | Indonesian rupiah |
| INA-CBG | Indonesia Case-Base Groups |
| Jasindo | Jasa Indonesia Company = The Indonesian Company for Insurance |
| Jamkesmas | Jaminan Kesehatan Masyarakat = Public health insurance |

| | |
|---|---|
| Jampelthas | Jaminan Pelayanan Thalasemia = Thalassemia insurance |
| Jampersal | Jaminan Persalinan = Maternity insurance |
| JKN | Jaminan Kesehatan Nasional = National health insurance |
| LOS | Length of stay |
| MOH | Ministry of Health = Kementerian Kesehatan |
| PHOJP | Public Health of Jakarta Province = Dinas Kesehatan Provinsi DKI Jakarta |
| RI | Republik Indonesia = The Republic of Indonesia |
| RM | Ringgit Malaysia |
| RSCM | Rumah Sakit Cipto Mangunkusumo = Cipto Mangunkusumo Hospital |
| SKTM | Surat Keterangan Tidak Mampu = Recommendation letter for borderline poor people |
| UNU | United Nations University |
| UPPJ | Unit Pelayanan Pasien Jaminan = Insurance Patient Services Unit |

# INTRODUCTION

## 1.1  Introduction

Health is one of the most important issues in every country in the world, including Indonesia. As a developing country, Indonesia has designated health as a priority and has introduced an excellent programme to improve its health care system. One of the health development goals outlined in the National Strategic Plan for Health through Regulation Number 40 of 2004 (The House of Representatives of the Republic of Indonesia 2004) is to provide financial protection and accessible health care for all Indonesians. This regulation is the main policy supporting the improvement of universal health coverage (UHC) initiatives to cover approximately 267.6 million people on 16,056 islands in 2016 (The Central Bureau Statistic 2017).

In 2000, the Jakarta provincial government launched the Gakin (Keluarga Maskin, or poor families) programme, known as the Jakarta Health Card (Kartu Jakarta Sehat (KJS)). The Gakin programme was a social health insurance programme only for

Jakarta residents that reimbursed health care providers using the fee-for-service (FFS) payment method (PHOJP 2009).

In 2008, the Indonesian government launched a national health insurance programme for poor people, previously called Jaminan Kesehatan Masyarakat (Jamkesmas) and now known as Jaminan Kesehatan Nasional (JKN/National Health Insurance). The Jamkesmas programme adopted the casemix method for hospital reimbursement with the National Drug Formulary under the Ministry of Health (MOH) (MOH 2010). The number of participants in Jamkesmas has gradually increased from 58.2 million people in 2008 and is expected to reach more than 270 million people in 2019 through the JKN programme (MOH 2017). To complete the social health insurance system in Indonesia, the MOH launched two additional social health insurance programmes, i.e., maternity insurance (Jaminan Persalinan, Jampersal) and thalassemia insurance (Jaminan Thalasemia, Jampelthas), both of which used the casemix method to reimburse providers in 2011 (MOH 2011).

From 2008 until 2012, two types of hospital payment methods were used in Indonesia's social health insurance programmes, i.e., the Gakin programme and the Jamkesmas programme. Gakin was operated by the Jakarta provincial government and used an FFS scheme for hospital reimbursement (PHOJP 2011), while the Jamkesmas programme, under the MOH, employed the casemix method. Both healthcare programmes covered the same benefit packages, including outpatient and inpatient services. Since 2012, the Gakin programme has changed its approach to hospital reimbursement by changing its payment method from FFS to casemix (PHOJP 2012). The benefit packages of the two programmes are similar, and patients in the Gakin programme have been incorporated into the casemix patient group. Therefore, 2011 was the last year in which the Gakin and Jamkesmas programmes had different reimbursement systems and patient group data.

In 2011, the Indonesian government launched the roadmap of achievement for the UHC programme. Presidential Regulation

Number 12 of 2013 officially designated the casemix payment method as the method for hospital reimbursement under the Indonesia UHC programme, and the FFS method has been eliminated. On January 1, 2014, the Indonesian government launched the UHC programme known as JKN (MOH 2014). A study should be conducted to assess whether choosing the casemix payment method for Indonesian UHC was a good strategic decision.

Regulations regarding charge reimbursement methods are important for the sustainability of a social insurance programme. JKN has been implemented with a limited budget but must cover a very large number of people; therefore, the provider payment method used in the programme should be carefully designed. The payment method should drive efficiency in hospitals, which are generally more expensive than primary health care. Selecting an appropriate provider payment method is one strategy that can be employed to control health care costs (Mathauer and Wittenbecher 2013).

A study should be conducted to assess whether choosing the casemix payment method for Indonesian UHC was a good strategic decision. It is important to study the implementation of the FFS and casemix approaches that were used in hospitals under the social health insurance scheme before 2012. The Gakin programme changed from FFS to casemix in 2012; thus, the year 2011 represents a period when the FFS and casemix methods had separate groups of patients, reimbursement charges, billing administrators, billing processes, social health security system regulations, and payers. This period represents a rare circumstance that cannot be repeated or created regularly; it is possible that the conditions of this period will occur only once.

This study assessed the casemix and FFS methods in natural conditions—without interventions from any stakeholders, including the researcher. Thus, these conditions are unique and have not occurred since in Indonesia. Using Indonesia's experiences, the researcher studied two familiar payment methods, i.e., FFS and casemix. This study is important because it describes the actual implementation of casemix and FFS as hospital reimbursement methods at the same time, in the same place, and using the same benefit packages for social health insurance in different groups of patients.

## 1.2    Statement of The Problems

UHC in Indonesia faces a large challenge to its goal of eventually covering all residents. The sustainability of this programme depends on many factors, one of which is the selection of an appropriate payment method. From 2008 until 2011, 2 payment methods were used for social health insurance, i.e., casemix and FFS

Table 1.1 Types of insurance and payments used for social health insurance in an Indonesian teaching hospital from 2008 to 2011

| Type of Health Insurance | Type of Payment |
|---|---|
| Gakin (Only for Jakarta residents) | Fee-for-service |
| Jamkesmas (Health security insurance) | Casemix |
| Jampersal (Maternity insurance) | Casemix |
| Jampelthas (Thalassemia insurance) | Casemix |

Source: Cipto Mangunkusumo Hospital 2011. The Annual Report

Presidential Regulation Number 12 of 2013 designated casemix as the official hospital reimbursement method under Indonesian UHC (MOH 2014). The design of the charge reimbursement method is one of the key factors for the sustainability of the UHC programme. The advantages and disadvantages of the charge reimbursement method should be considered carefully. Due to the limited source of funding, the implementation of the method will have an impact on the efficient use of available resources.

A study should be conducted to assess whether choosing the casemix payment method for Indonesian UHC was a good strategic decision. This study aims to determine why the casemix method was chosen for hospital reimbursement instead of the FFS method. This study will also attempt to determine the advantages of casemix implementation in medical care and billing systems for hospital reimbursement under the social health insurance system.

## 1.3    Justification for The Study

The Jakarta provincial government selected the FFS method for the Gakin programme (Keluarga Maskin or poor family), which had two groups of participants, i.e., Gakin Card participants and Surat Keterangan Tidak Mampu (SKTM/recommendation letter for borderline poor people) participants. The Gakin and SKTM patient groups represent the samples for the FFS payment method and are called the Gakin programme in this study.

The MOH selected the casemix reimbursement method for the National Health Financing system, which consisted of public health insurance for the poor (Jamkesmas), maternity insurance (Jampersal), and thalassemia insurance (Jampelthas). These programmes, together called Jamkesmas, represent the samples for the casemix payment method.

In 2012, the reimbursement method used by the Gakin programme was changed from the FFS method to the casemix scheme. The policy underlying the Gakin programme has been changed to Jamkesmas, and Gakin programme participants have been incorporated into the casemix group. Therefore, 2011 was the last year in which the Gakin programme and the Jamkesmas programme had different reimbursement systems. Accordingly, our study collected data for the year 2011, as the patient groups and reimbursement data for the FFS and casemix methods were still entirely different the during this year.

The largest national referral and main teaching hospital in Jakarta, Indonesia, was chosen as the site of this study. This hospital provided health care for a very large number of patients using the FFS and casemix payment methods and served patients from all the provinces in Indonesia, thus becoming the largest national referral hospital in Indonesia. The hospital served as a health provider for all health security insurance in Indonesia, including the Gakin and Jamkesmas programmes.

The hospital management information system (HMIS) was just beginning to be built in 2008, so the hospital data were reported semi-manually, and electronic health records (EHRs) were not integrated between medical service units. The data were not complete and were scattered across several service units. Therefore, the data were collected manually from patient medical records, EHRs, patient reports, registration records, and financial reports. Due to the very large number of patients, it is possible that many samples were not collected for this study.

Considering the huge number of patients during 2011 which needed longer time for collecting data manually from the patient medical records; semi manually for the very huge number of hospitals claim data, and the limited budget and time, the researcher determined that the data collection for this study was only data in the year of 2011.

## 1.4    Significance of The Study

This study assessed the implementation of the casemix and FFS methods under natural conditions—without intervention from any stakeholders, including the researcher. The Gakin programme changed from FFS to casemix in 2012; thus, the year 2011 represents a period when the FFS and casemix methods had separate groups of patients, reimbursement charges, billing administrators, billing processes, regulations, and payers.

The results of this study are very important for supporting Indonesian UHC—the JKN programme—which was established in January 2014. The sustainability of the JKN programme should be supported by designing and regulating a good provider payment method in Indonesia. Inappropriate decisions or regulations could cause a lack of funding or inefficiencies that could eventually terminate the JKN programme.

Through this study, the results of comparisons between the two reimbursement schemes can offer feedback for decision makers and policy makers (e.g., the MOH) for developing the social health care system. Good policies are important to supporting the achievement of the UHC system, which provided health insurance for approximately 171.9 million people or 64.23% of the Indonesian population in 2016; the system continues to improve and aims to reach its target of covering all Indonesian people (more than 270 million people) in 2019 (DJSN 2012).

This study provides empirical evidence to determine whether Presidential Regulation Number 12 of 2013, which designated the casemix payment method as the official hospital reimbursement method, was a good decision. A study is needed to develop appropriate recommendations for improving the hospital reimbursement system and supporting UHC in Indonesia. A comparison between the casemix and FFS methods shows the advantages and disadvantages of the two methods for medical care and financing.

The study results can be used by hospital management or organizations involved in Indonesian UHC. Hospital managers will be enriched by knowledge of the hospital reimbursement method under the social health security system, thus improving their understanding of casemix as the official hospital reimbursement method for UHC. The study includes many sub-studies, i.e., analyses of medical services, unnecessary admissions, the billing process, the cost of the billing process, and claims paid by payers. Hospital directors or managers should make very good strategic decisions or implement regulations to increase efficiency without decreasing the quality of health care. This study offers very important considerations for hospital managers before their hospitals join the UHC programme as health providers.

This study enriches the understanding of clinicians and hospital staff about the casemix and FFS methods for hospital reimbursement. These groups gain an understanding of what they should do to provide medical services for patients under both payment methods. This study also offers feedback and recommendations for improving services and behaviour and for preventing overtreatment and over prescribing.

For academic researchers and health practices, this study is an exploration of Indonesia's experiences during a period when the country was preparing for UHC. This study records very important knowledge for academics and scientists and enriches the knowledge base regarding the impact of the casemix and FFS methods of hospital reimbursement. This study also demonstrates the benefits and disadvantages of casemix and FFS implementation, particularly the cost of the billing process, which has very rarely been reported elsewhere. Comparing the cost of the billing process and studying the billing process and unnecessary admissions are not easily achieved because data are rarely available. In addition, there are more studies on medical care than on the cost of the billing process. For many researchers, the cost of the billing process is less familiar than the cost of medical care. This study enriches the knowledge of researchers regarding casemix and FFS implementation. Thus, all the study results can be used as a reference in other academic research and can be explored in further studies.

## 1.5   Research Objectives

### 1.5.1 General Objectives

This study aimed to examine the impact of the implementation of the casemix method for hospital reimbursement scheme of FFS and casemix methods in a teaching hospital in Indonesia.

## 1.5.2 Specific Objectives

1. To describe the social demography and classification of primary diagnoses for patients whose costs were reimbursed using the casemix system under the social health insurance scheme.

2. To determine and compare the impact of patients' hospital charges and length of stay (LOS) for the casemix and FFS methods.

3. To compare the impact of rates of unnecessary patient admission for the casemix and FFS methods.

4. To analyse the impact of cost of the billing process for patients whose costs were reimbursed through the casemix method and the FFS method.

5. To compare the impact of percentage of patients' claims reimbursed under the casemix and FFS methods.

6. To compare perception of the billing processes used for the casemix and FFS methods.

## 1.6   Research Questions

1. Does the casemix method have a shorter LOS than the FFS method in this teaching hospital?

2. Does the casemix system have lower charges than the FFS method in this teaching hospital?

3. Does the casemix method have a lower rate of unnecessary admission than the FFS method in this teaching hospital?

4. Does the casemix method have lower billing process costs than the FFS method in this teaching hospital?

5. Does the casemix system have a higher percentage of claims reimbursment than the FFS method in this teaching hospital?

6. Is the billing process for reimbursement under the FFS method more complex than that under the casemix method in this teaching hospital?

## 1.7   Research Hypotheses

1. Patients whose costs are reimbursed using the casemix method has shorter lengths of stay than those whose costs are reimbursed using the fee-for-service method.
2. Hospital charges under the fee-for-service method are higher than those under the casemix payment method.
3. The rate of unnecessary admission is lower among patients whose costs are reimbursed using the casemix method than among those whose costs are reimbursed using the fee-for-service method.
4. The cost of the billing process for patients under the casemix reimbursement method is lower than that for patients under the fee-for-service method.
5. The percentage of claims reimbursed under the casemix method is higher than that under the fee-for-service method.
6. The billing process for reimbursement under the fee-for-service method is more complex than that under the casemix method.

## 1.8   Conceptual Framework of The Study

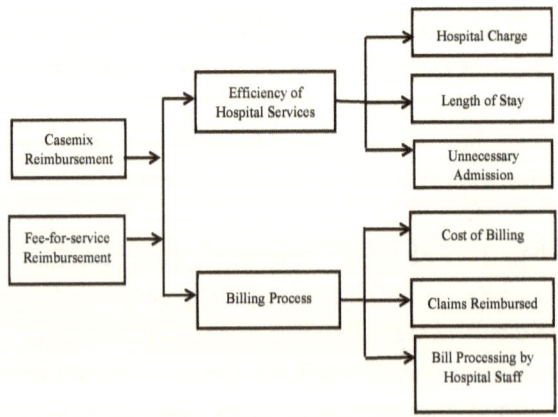

Figure 1.1 Conceptual framework of the study
Scheme of Reimbursement and Impact Assessment

To fulfil the objectives of the study, the conceptual frame work was designed to compare 2 types of hospital reimbursement payment methods under social health insurance programmes, i.e., the FFS and casemix methods. The framework included two important aspects: the efficiency of hospital services and the billing process used by hospital staff.

The comparison of efficiency was assessed based on hospital charges for outpatient and inpatient services, LOS and the rate of unnecessary admissions for patients whose costs were reimbursed using the FFS method and for patients whose costs were reimbursed using the casemix method. Hospital charge and LOS are the two main variables in health care expenditures (WHO 2010). LOS, in conjunction with hospital charge and health care expenditures, reflects the efficiency of hospital services. The comparisons of hospital charge and LOS between the two reimbursement systems were conducted with the 5 most common primary diagnoses. Unnecessary admission cases, which reflect inefficiency in health care expenditures (Amaro 2010) were compared between the two payment methods. Efficiency can be determined by measuring and comparing average LOS (ALOS) (Aljunid 2012) and rates of unnecessary admission (Amaro 2010).

For the billing process analysis, this study assessed the cost of the billing process, hospital claims reimbursed and bill processing by hospital staff members. The cost of the billing process determines the cost of one patient's bill for the casemix and FFS methods. A lower cost of billing decreases the operational cost of hospital management. To increase knowledge about the billing process in a teaching hospital, a survey on perceptions of the billing process used for the FFS and casemix methods was conducted among billing administrators via a questionnaire (MOH 2011; PHOJP 2011). The billing process is very important for maintaining a hospital's cash flow. Cashflow in health care is based on revenue, which is mostly earned by rendering services to patients (Finkler, et al 2013). Payment for these services influences a hospital's cash flow. Therefore, the percentage of claims paid by payers was calculated and compared for the two payment methods. The cash flow of a hospital is very important, and the hospital's claim process plays an important role in promoting the sustainability of patient care and hospital activities (Green 2016).

## 1.9   Definition of Terms

1. Fee-for-service (FFS) is retrospective payment to a provider for each act or service rendered (Cashin 2015).
2. FFS is a payment method that uses FFS for reimbursement.
3. Casemix is a payment method that uses the casemix system for reimbursement.
4. Casemix is a classification of patient treatment episodes designed to create classes that are relatively homogenous with respect the resources used and that contain patients with similar clinical characteristics (Palmer G and Reid B 2001).
5. The Gakin programme (Keluarga Maskin/poor family) is a health insurance programme for the poor residents of Jakarta province; the programme used the FFS method for hospital reimbursement (PHOJP 2011).
6. Jaminan Kesehatan Masyarakat (Jamkesmas) is a public health insurance programme under the social health insurance programme through the Ministry of Health (MOH); Jamkesmas uses the casemix system for hospital reimbursement and consists of Jamkesmas, maternity insurance (JaminanPersalinan/Jampersal) and thalassemia insurance (Jaminan Thalasemia/Jampelthas) (MOH 2011).
7. The costs for patients under the Gakin programme were reimbursed using the FFS method in 2011.
8. The costs for patients under Jamkesmas programme were reimbursed using the casemix method in 2011.

9. The social demography information includes age, gender and referral area (MOH 2016).

10. Primary diagnose is the condition diagnosed at the end of an episode of health care that is primarily responsible for the patient's need for treatment or investigation and is determined to have been mainly responsible for the health care episode.

11. Hospital tariff was the payment received by hospitals on the medical service or non-medical service that were done to the patients (MOH 2015).

12. Length of stay (LOS) is the period of time a patient remains in a hospital or other health care facility as an inpatient (WHO 2010).

13. An unnecessary admission consists of a person who is admitted to a hospital as an inpatient and spends one day or less in the hospital, even though his/her condition did not warrant admission (Means 2016).

14. Cost is all resources sacrificed to produce or consume one commodity or product in products or services (Finkler 2013).

15. The billing process is the steps of the procedure used to prepare a patient's bill for health care from admission until discharge (Green and Rowell 2015)

16. The complexity of the billing process is driven by the steps of the procedure that require more resources and time and additional activities.

17. The cost of the billing process is the cost that is needed to process patient bills and patient claims that are delivered to payers.

18. The human resources cost is the cost for employees such as wages, renumeration, overtimes fees, and insurance (RSCM 2017).

19. The stationery cost is the cost of paper, printer paper, computer ink, copies, computer maintenance, and containers for documents (RSCM 2017).

20. The transportation cost is the cost for delivering billing claims from the hospital to the payer's office and the cost of transportation for verifiers (RSCM 2017).
21. The hospital claim reimbursed is the payment of the hospital claims that are verified and approved by the payers (MOH 2018).

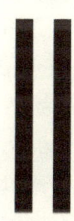

# LITERATURE REVIEW

## 2.1 Health Insurance in Indonesia

The Indonesian government began to introduce the principle of health insurance in 1947—two years after Indonesia won its independence. Unfortunately, the security situation after independence was very unstable, which resulted in health insurance not being adopted or being developed well at that time. In 1960, the Indonesian government tried to introduce another health insurance programme through the Basic Health Care Act of 1960, but due to socio-economic difficulties, the programme could not be implemented. In 1967, the Indonesian government issued a health financing programme that was similar to a health maintenance organization (HMO) and implemented the Basic Health Care Act of 1960 (Jasindo 2012). In 1995, PT Askes was founded as a state-owned enterprise to manage the government's basic health care programme. The number of hospital providers and benefits increased gradually. In 2000, Askes declared its vision as a specialist and as the government's health insurance provider. In late 2004, Askes announced that 2% of the insurance fee would be subsidized by the government, while 2% would be paid by employees (Askes 2012).

In the 1900s, many provincial governments attempted to improve health care for poor families. One of those provincial governments was the Jakarta provincial government, which assisted the poor through its Gakin (Keluarga Maskin or poor family) programme. In the 2000s, the Gakin programme was expanded to cover borderline poor people using the Surat Keterangan Tidak Mampu (SKTM or recommendation letter for borderline poor people) letter. The Gakin programme was made available only to residents of Jakarta and was funded by the provincial government of Jakarta using the fee-for-service (FFS) method for hospital reimbursement. To control costs, the Gakin programme had an essential services package (Paket Pelayanan Essensial (PPE)) that had a maximum reimbursement of up to IDR 100,000,000 (PHOJP 2009) and used generic drugs (MOH 2010). From 2012 until 2013, the Gakin programme gradually reformed its reimbursement method from FFS to casemix and was renamed the Kartu Jakarta Sehat (KJS/Jakarta Health Card) programme (PHOJP 2012).

The casemix system was implemented for the first time in Indonesia through the Jaminan Kesehatan Masyarakat (Jamkesmas, public health insurance) programme in September 2008 by the Ministry of Health (MOH). This payment model was used initially in 15 national hospitals as a pilot project and was then expanded to cover all provincial and district hospitals in Indonesia. The Jamkesmas programme provided health insurance for poor and borderline poor people. This programme was financed by taxes allocated from the central government, and it did not require any insurance contribution or cost sharing on the part of the programme beneficiaries. In 2009, many provincial governments in Indonesia launched Jaminan Kesehatan Daerah (Jamkesda or district health insurance) programmes, which used casemix for hospital reimbursement. All the Jamkesda programmes gradually joined the Jamkesmas programme in using the casemix method. Later in 2011, the MOH launched two new health programmes, i.e., Jaminan Persalinan (Jampersal, maternity insurance) and Jaminan Pelayanan Thalasemia (Jampelthas, thalassemia insurance), and incorporated casemix as their charge reimbursement method for hospitals (MOH 2011).

In 2004, the Indonesian Parliament approved the National Social Security System (Sistem Jaminan Sosial Nasional) through Law Number 44 of 2004, which appointed Badan Penyelenggara Jaminan Sosial (BPJS, the Public Health Social Insurance Implementing Body) as the legal institution responsible for implementing the social security system (BPJS 2016). One strategic programme of the BPJS was the implementation of universal health coverage (UHC) in 2014 using the casemix method for hospital reimbursement, as stipulated in Presidential Regulation Number 12 of 2013. On January 1, 2014, the Indonesian government declared the Jaminan Kesehatan Nasional (JKN/National Health Insurance) programme to be the Indonesian UHC programme; it is designed to gradually provide all Indonesian citizens with health insurance. Currently, all social health insurance schemes in Indonesia are under one programme, the JKN (MOH 2014).

To support the UHC programme, the Indonesian government issued Presidential Regulation Number 77 of 2012, which states that health expenditures are part of the national health system. In Indonesia, health expenditures rapidly improved following this change in the government's health policy. In addition, Indonesia's health expenditures represent only 3.8% of GDP and are lower than those of several Association of Southeast Asian Nations (ASEAN) countries.

Table 2.1 Health expenditures of several ASEAN countries in 2016

| Country | Health expenditures per capita (US$) | Share of GDP (%) | Social health insurance share (%) |
|---|---|---|---|
| Indonesia | 126 | 3.8 | 13.0 |
| Malaysia | 456 | 4.2 | 0.6 |
| Philippines | 135 | 4.7 | 14.0 |
| Thailand | 360 | 6.5 | 5.1 |
| Vietnam | 142 | 7.1 | 24.1 |

Source: MOH 2016. The Indonesia Health Profile.

Since 2014, the number of participants in the UHC programme, which covers poor people, government employees, private company workers, informal sector workers and common people, has increased gradually. Only 13% of GDP is used to cover premiums for poor people and premium subsidies for government employees under the UHC programme.

Table 2.2 Number of participants in the universal health coverage programme in Indonesia from 2014 to 2016

| Year | Number of participants | Participants as a percentage of Indonesia's population (%) |
|------|------------------------|-----------------------------------------------------------|
| 2014 | 133,425,052 | 51.8 |
| 2015 | 156,790,287 | 60.8 |
| 2016 | 171,939,254 | 66.7 |

Source: MOH 2016. The Indonesia Health Profile.

The number of UHC participants increases yearly, and the Indonesia government still has ambitions to cover all Indonesian citizens by 2019 according to the Road Map of Indonesian Universal Health Coverage (DJSN 2012).

## 2.2 Provider Payment Mechanism

Health is a state of complete physical, mental, and social wellbeing and is not merely the absence of disease or infirmity (WHO 2010). Health care systems in many developing countries have similar challenges in areas such as efficiency and provider payment systems (Mills 2005). Provider payment systems can be useful for improving the development of a health system and for achieving health policy objectives by encouraging access to health services for patients, promoting high-quality care and improving equality while promoting the effective and efficient use of the resources and, where appropriate, cost containment (Berenson 2016).

Provider payment mechanisms are very important for health care insurance. Provider payment mechanisms influence quality of care, cost containment and the provision of services such as curative vs. preventive and basic vs. advanced health services. Those influences have impacts on the efficiency of health expenditures and the viability of the health financing scheme. Poor provider payment mechanisms create challenges in health financing schemes and result in high levels of inefficiency (Palmer and Reid 2001).

Two types of provider payment methods are used in many countries (Aljunid 2012, Hicks 2014):

1. Retrospective payment: payments are made or agreed upon after the provision of services.

   Example: Fee-for-service (FFS),

2. Prospective payment: payments are made or agreed upon in advance before the provision of services.

   Examples: Capitation, global budget, line-item budget and casemix.

According to the objectives of this study, the literature review presents the FFS payment method as a retrospective payment method and the casemix method as a prospective payment method. Both of these provider payment mechanisms have been implemented in Indonesia

Meanwhile in prospective payment, capitation (per capita) is defined that providers are paid a fixed amount in advance to provide a defined package of services for each enrolled individual for a fixed period of time. Capitation is useful for management capacity of the purchaser, invreasing competition, strengthening primary care, cost control and health promotion. The lack of capitation payment method create the manipulative data for increasing the fund, underprovide services, increasing the referrals to the higher health providers level, select the healthier enrolees for less costly.

The Global budget payment method is defined that health providers receive a fixed amount for a specified period to cover aggregate expenditures to provide an agreed-upon set of services. The budget can be spent flexibly and is not tied to line items. This payment method has the competition among providers is not possible or not an objective, cost control is a top priority. But, global budgets are formed based on inputs can underprovide services and increase referrals to other providers. If global budgets are formed based on volume can increase the number of services and referrals to other providers. Mechanism exists to improve efficiency but may need to be combined with other incentives.

In line-item budget, health providers receive a fixed amount for a specified period to cover specific input expenses (e.g., personnel, medicines, utilities). The budget is not flexible, and expenditure must follow line items. Management capacity of the purchaser and providers is low, cost control is a top priority; financial management and monitoring are weak. This payment method has underprovide services, increase referrals to other providers, increase inputs, spend all remaining funds by the end of the budget year. No incentive or mechanism to improve efficiency.

In per diem, hospitals are paid a fixed amount per day for each admitted patient. The per diem rate may vary by department, patient, clinical characteristics, or other factors. Increase the number of bed-days, which may lead to excessive admissions and lengths of hospital stays. The lack of this payment method increase inputs per bed-day, which may improve the inefficiency of the input mix or possibly reduce quality (Cashin 2015).

## 2.2.1 Fee-for-service (FFS)

FFS is one of the most popular payment methods in health care systems. FFS involves traditional provider reimbursement for each individual service provided by the hospital and usually uses the provider's charge. Fee-for-service is defined that providers are paid for each individual service delivered. Fees or tariffs are fixed in advance for each service or bundle services. FFS payments reimburse providers for delivering individual items, such as doctor consultations, X-ray tests, surgical operations, and other services. The FFS method also covers itemized charges for all medical procedures or treatments and drugs (Beik 2015).

The FFS payment method can be further divided into 2 subgroups (Langenbrunner, Cheryl and O'Dougherty 2009):

1.  Fee-for-service without a fixed fee schedule.

This FFS payment represents the traditional type of FFS, which is an open-ended fee charged by a doctor according to the market. Providers are permitted to bill purchasers for all costs incurred to provide each service. Indonesia implemented this form of FFS for its Gakin programme (PHOJP 2009).

2.  Fee-for service with a fixed fee schedule and bundling of services.

Fee-for-service with a fixed fee schedule and the bundling of services came into existence with the establishment of health insurance schemes. Services are bundled, and the provider is paid a fixed fee for the services. The provider has an incentive to increase the number of services overall for an encounter and to reduce the inputs used for each service. This form of FFS was used in Indonesia for the Askes programme until 2013 (Askes 2012) when the programme was changed to use casemix for UHC.

The FFS payment method has some advantages:

1.  The FFS method can be easily developed and implemented, as in the community financing schemes used for their start-ups (Boachie 2014).

2.  The FFS payment method more accurately reflects the work performed and the effort expended. This method of payment encourages providers to work longer hours or deliver more services (Langenbrunner, Cheryl and O'Dougherty 2009).
3.  The FFS method improves access and utilization for underserved areas (MOH of NZ 2015).
4.  The FFS method can be designed to encourage the provision of cost-effective services (Moreno-Serra and Wagstaff 2009).

Studies have revealed the disadvantages of the FFS payment method:

1.  In most countries, FFS can potentially result in a large explosion of expenditures and uncontrolled outcomes (Wiessenberger & Thommen & Schuetz et al 2013).
2.  FFS incurs high administrative costs for both providers and insurers/payers. This result occurs partly because every service and procedure must be billed. For this reason, FFS is considered good for providers' internal efficiency and poor for social efficiency from the consumer's point of view (Wiessenberger & Thommen & Schuetz et al 2013).
3.  FFS payment method correlates with a pronounced increase in health expenditures, high operational costs, inefficiency and cost escalation (Limwattananon and Tangcharoensathien 2010).
4.  FFS as a method for health reimbursement has a higher total medicine cost for uninsured patients than other payment methods. The FFS system has been found to result in the prescription of more medicines per visit and in higher costs in the private sector than in the public sector (Langenbrunner, Cheryl and O'Dougherty 2009).
5.  The FFS system is the most uncontrollable payment method and drives the use of services that increase moral hazard and inefficiency in health expenditures (Green 2016).

The billing process under the FFS method used a billing slip for every procedure and hospital care service. All billings were calculated into the hospital's claim and then delivered to the payer.

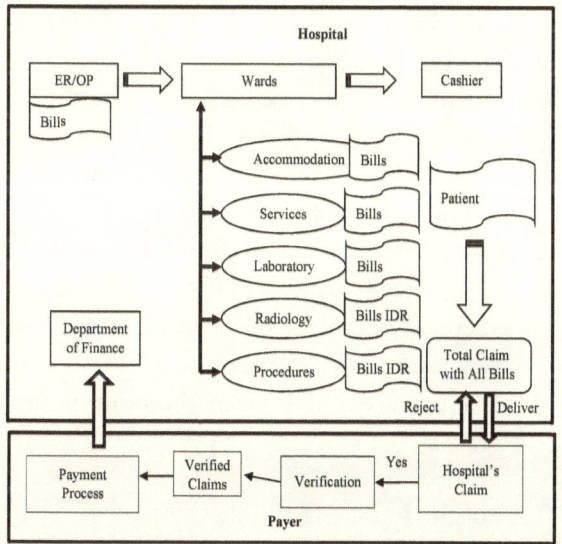

Figure 2.1 Billing process of the fee-for-service payment method
Source: The Public Health of Jakarta Province. 2011.
The Technical Guideline of The Social Health Security
and Disaster System in Jakarta Province 2011.

For each patient, bills were generated for every medical care or service, then all bills were calculated into a single patient bill when the patient was discharged from the hospital. All patient bills were collected into a total hospital claim for one month. The total hospital claim was then delivered to the payer with supporting documents. If those documented claims were approved by the payer, then the claim was paid to the hospital. If the claim was rejected and not approved with notification, the claim documents were sent back to the hospital. The hospital could complete or revise the claim documents based on the notification and then send the revised claim back to the payer. The payer verified the claims and paid the claim amounts to the hospital.

The regulation for submitting a hospital's claim to a payer required the claim for each patient's bill to be accompanied by many documents for payment verification (PHOJP 2011):

1. Copy of the patient's membership card for the Gakin programme.
2. For patients who were not Gakin members:

   a. Copy of the patient's SKTM (recommendation letter for borderline poor people).
   b. Verification results from the officers of Public Health of Jakarta Province (PHOJP). This letter verified whether the patient was insured 100%, insured 50% or not insured by Jakarta province.
   c. A letter of domicile from the head of the patient's village.

3. Copy of the Indonesia Family Card.
4. National Identity Card.

   a. Copy of the Indonesia National Identity Card for adult patients 17 years of age and older.
   b. Copy of the Indonesia National Identity Card for the parents of paediatric patients.

5. A referral letter from the patient's primary health care provider.
6. A referral letter from the hospital (if available).
7. A Letter of Health Service Insurance approved by PHOJP officers in the hospital.
8. All the bills for each individual health care service such as doctor consultations, medical health officer consultations, medical procedures, diagnostic procedures, drugs and pharmaceutical care, wards, and blood bags.
9. Doctor's requirement for medical procedures or diagnostic procedures.

10. The results of medical surgeries.
11. Approval from PHOJP officers for each expensive medical and diagnostic procedure, drug and pharmaceutical service.
12. The doctor's instructions for discharged patients.
13. PHOJP officers' approval for and determination on cost sharing for the patient's total bill.
14. An approval letter for catastrophic coverage up to IDR 100,000,000 from the PHOJP.
15. Bank payment for cost sharing for SKTM patients.
16. Death certificate (for patients who died in the hospital).
17. Medical chart (if available).

These documents were prepared, and the originals were sent to the payer, while copies were made for the hospital's archives. All the documents were delivered to the payer's office with a summary report and a cover letter from the hospital's president director. The summary document and the cover letter from the president director were archived by the department of finance in the hospital.

### 2.2.2 Casemix

The history of casemix saw its earliest formal developments in the 1960s at Oxford University. Professor Martin Feldstein found that the types of patients treated by a hospital had a large influence on the hospital's costs. This work on casemix continued at Yale University around 1967 by Professor Robert Fetter, Professor John Thompson, and colleagues. The Yale group was responsible for the development of the first diagnostic-related group (DRG) and for creating a better understanding of the issues and concepts associated with casemix (Green 2016).

In the early 1980s, the Health Care Financing Administration (HCFA) funded the Yale group to develop an improved version of DRG that would then include basic payments to hospitals from the federal government for Medicare inpatients. HCFA has continued to fund the development of new versions of the DRG. In the initial period, there were only 383 DRGs. In the United States, Medicare used fix prices with 474 DRGs in 1983. In 1985, there were several recalculations of the casemix index (Quinn 2015).

Table 2.3 History of the casemix system

| Year | Country | Casemix Development |
|------|---------|---------------------|
| 1967 | England | Professor Robert Fetter, Professor John Thompson, and colleagues (Yale group) created the first DRG |
| 1980s | United Kingdom | Improve 492 DRGs |
| 1983 | USA | Using HCFA-DRG |
| 1985 | Portugal | The first country outside the UK to use casemix |
| 1992 | Australia | Aus-DRG |
| 1997 | South Korea | K-DRG |
| 2002 | Malaysia | MY-DRG |
| 2003 | Japan | J-DRG |
| 2003 | Germany | G-DRG |
| 2008 | Indonesia | INA-CBGs |

Source: Aljunid 2012, MOH 2016; Adams (2012).

The casemix system is defined as a classification of patient treatment episodes to create classes that are relatively homogenous with respect to resources used and that contain patients with similar clinical characteristics (Palmer and Reid 2001). Casemix has two main objectives: to categorize patients' common clinical attributes and similar output utilization patterns into clinically meaningful groups and to provide a means for examining the products of the hospital (Fetter and Freeman 1980).

Two main components of the casemix payment method are disease classification and cost analysis (Aljunid 2012, Adams 2012):

## 1. Disease classification

Diseases are grouped by diagnoses, which are determined based on clinical and resource homogeneity. All primary and secondary diagnoses are coded using the International Classification of Diseases, Tenth Revision (ICD-10), while the International Classification of Diseases, Ninth Revision, Clinical Modification (ICD-9 CM) is used for procedure codes. Many variables are needed to build a DRG or case-base group (CBG) such as patient's identity, date of birth, age, gender, type of care, date of admission, date of discharge, LOS, discharge status, primary diagnosis, secondary diagnosis, and procedures and the body weight of newborn babies (in grams) aged 0-28 days.

The primary diagnosis is defined as the condition diagnosed at the end of an episode of health care that is primarily responsible for the patient's need for treatment or investigation and is determined to have been mainly responsible for the health care episode. If there is more than one such condition, the condition that is held most responsible for the greatest use of resources should be selected. The rules for selecting the primary diagnosis include diagnoses at the end of an episode of healthcare, the greatest utilization of resources during the patient's stay and LOS justification (Buck 2012). The secondary diagnosis is a diagnosis that eithers co-exists with the primary diagnosis at the time of admission or appears during the episode of care. Secondary diagnoses are known as comorbidities and complications. Comorbidities are conditions that exist prior to admission, and complications are conditions that occur in the hospital (Adams 2012, MOH 2014).

Primary procedures are related to the primary diagnosis and require the most utilization of resources or the longest LOS. Secondary procedures are all the significant medical procedures performed for inpatients and outpatients that require special equipment or are completed by trained and experienced staff members (Adams 2012).

Clinical characteristics and resources are correlated in the clinical pathway. The clinical pathway is a multidisciplinary plan of care based on the best clinical practice for specified groups of patients with a particular diagnosis and is designed to minimize delays, optimize resource utilization and maximize quality of care (Campbell & Cegolon et al 2016). A very large number of clinical pathways exist in the hospital, and in the casemix system, hospital management must select cases for clinical pathways based on aspects such as common conditions, high volume, high costs and predictable outcomes.

Clinical pathways support casemix implementation by reducing variations in care, increasing the homogeneity of cases and improving the quality of casemix data, casemix cost analysis, and casemix parameters. Clinical pathways can be an internal control on the providers' health care expenditures, and clinical pathways are used as tools to monitor and evaluate health care expenditures for health services (Rozany & Yuliansyah and Susilo 2017, MOH 2014).

Clinical pathways provide a guideline for single-episode charges under casemix; a single episode starts when a patient is hospitalized and continues until the patient is discharged from the hospital. Single-episode charges consist of all the medical treatments and procedures, diagnostic procedures, pharmaceutical services, consultations and hospital accommodation utilized during a patient's stay in the hospital (Fetter and Freeman 1980, MOH 2014). The single-episode charge approach is a good system for performing internal cost control within hospital management and for reducing patients' medical costs (Adams 2012). Single-episode hospital charges under casemix create more systematic cost control and prevent overprescribing, overtreatment, over use of procedures, and other unnecessary actions (Aljunid 2012), and using the single-episode charge approach in casemix systems improves efficiency in referral hospitals (Wibowo 2013).

Level of severity is determined by comorbidities and complications. Comorbidities are conditions that accompany the main diagnosis and require treatment and care in addition to the treatment provided for the condition for which the patient was admitted, i.e., hypertension, diabetes mellitus (Buck 2012). Complications are diseases that appear during an episode of care due to a pre-existing condition or that arise from the care the patient receives, for example, post-operative wound infection (MOH 2016; Adams 2012).

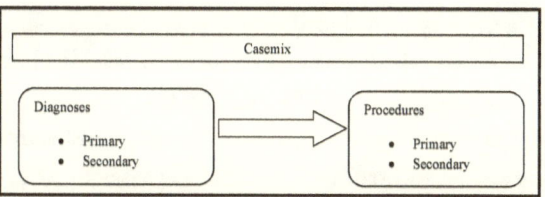

Figure 2.2 Relationship between diagnoses and
procedures in the casemix method
Source: MOH 2016; Adam 2012.

## 2. Cost analysis

Casemix uses top-down costing and activity-based costing (ABC). The ABC method is typically used for specific procedures. Top-down costing uses several indicators to separate all overhead costs into intermediate service overhead and final service overhead. Top-down costing starts with the total expenditures, then divides these by a measure of total output to determine an "average" cost per patient per visit per day or per admission. Top-down costing accurately determines the cost of achieving programme outputs or results by allocating all the costs of running a hospital to departments providing the final output of the hospital (Shepard & Hodgkin & Anthony 2000).

Casemix offers various negative incentives for providers (Boachie 2014):

- "Code creep", in which the provider classifies patients into groups coded for high reimbursement;

- Cost shifting, in which the provider shifts the patterns of care and costs to non-casemix patients and casemix settings, resulting in an unchanged total cost to the purchaser;
- Increases in unnecessary admissions and readmissions—in Hungary, Russia, and many other countries, the number of admissions increased significantly after a case-based system was introduced;
- Underproviding services or prematurely discharging and admitting patients—in such cases, costs are shifted to outpatient services, home service care, and nursing home care. The interruption of care decreases its effectiveness.

The FFS method uses every transaction in the medical services. Under the FFS method, hospital charges increase the hospital's profit significantly as the volume of medical care transactions increases. The higher the volume is, the higher the profit. However, under the casemix method, the volume of transactions does not always increase profit. Profit is obtained through efficiency in medical expenses, which should be controlled under total expenses (Dewar 2017).

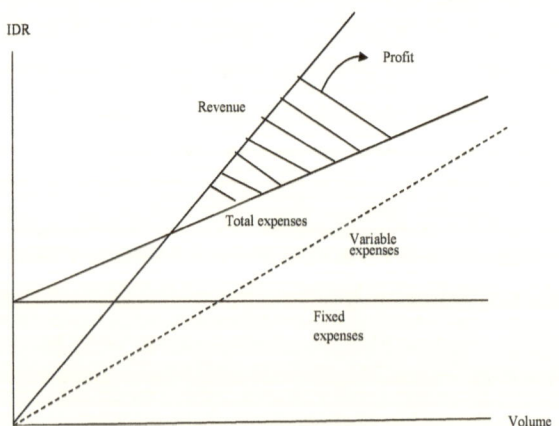

Figure 2.3 Economics of per case payment
Source: Wendel, J. O'donohue, W. Serratt, T 2014

A major advantage of the casemix method is that it removes the economic incentives for a hospital to provide as many items of service as possible (as with FFS) and to keep the patient in the hospital as long as possible (as with per diem). Average LOS (ALOS) typically decreases under casemix (Timbie & Bogart & Damberg et al 2017).

The casemix payment method has many advantages for hospital charge reimbursement:

1.  Improving the efficiency of services and reducing costs:

    — Reducing LOS (Mahendradhata and Trisnantoro 2017, Sulku 2011, Moshiri 2010, Carek and Boggan and Geesey 2008, Taheri 2001, Coelho and Fernandes et al 2010)
    — Identifying unnecessary hospitalizations (Ham and Candace 2010, Stranges and Stocks 2008, Richard and Pitluk 2008)
    — Analysing the productivity of employees (Green 2016)
    — Reducing re-admissions (Nevola & Pace & Karim et al 2016)
    — Reducing unnecessary admissions (Amaro 2010, Louis & Taroni & Melotti et al 2008)
    — Reducing hospital charges (Mathauer and Wittenbecher 2013, Yip & Hsiao et al 2010, Zhang 2010)

2.  Improving quality of care:

    — Reducing the number of severe illness (Wibowo 2013)
    — Improving the IT system used for medical services (Scheller-Kreinsen & Quentin & Busse 2011, Busse & Geissler & Quentin & Wiley 2011)
    — Improving mortality rates (Weissenberger, Thommen, and Schuetz 2013)
    — Improving the quality of hospital care (Anderson and Ikegami 2011)

3. Improving the quality of medical documents (Busse et al 2013, Medici and Murray 2010)
4. Reducing the number of documents for billing (Buck 2012)

## 2.2.3 Impact of The Payment Method Implementation

### a. Hospital tariff

In the FFS method, hospital tariffs vary among patients, as every patient receivescare according to their individual needs (Cashin 2015) in which the providers (hospitals) are paid for each individual service provided (Li et al 2015). Overtreatment and overmedication are disadvantages of the FFS method, and they lead to high operational costs, inefficiency, and cost escalation (Campbell et al 2016). The FFS method leads to a pronounced increase in the volume of services (Hopfe et al 2016). The FFS method uses per procedure invoicing, which tends to lack cost controls and increases the costs for patients as well as increasing moral hazard in various countries (Medici & Murray 2010).

In a casemix implementation, one-episode hospital tariffs create more systematic cost control and prevent over prescription, overtreatment, unnecessary procedures, and other unnecessary actions (Ham et al 2010. Casemix tariff is associated with reduced hospital tariffs (Stranges et a 2010) reduced cost (Li et al 2015) and reducing hospital charges (Mathauer and Wittenbecher 2013, Yip & Hsiao et al 2010, Zhang 2010)

### b. Length of stay (LOS)

The FFS method correlates with unnecessarily and inappropriately long LOS (Coelho & Fernandes et al 2010). Also, FFS correlates with a pronounced increase in the volume of services and overall expenditures and unnecessarily long LOS and this situation increasingly creates moral hazards in many countries and increases inefficiency in services (Murakami & Lorenzoni 2015).

In contrast with the FFS method, the casemix method implemented the one-episode charge approach to control costs per patient (Kim & Kim 2017). Casemix reduced the patient's medical cost and LOS and speeding up the turnover of hospital beds (Wang & Hellers et al 2017).

### c. Unnecessary admission

Unnecessary admission is one health cost attributable to inefficiency; moreover, the hospital tariff of a national referral hospital, the site investigated in this study, is more expensive than those of the lower-tier health facilities. However, the previous lower-tier hospitals, which referred the unnecessarily admitted patients to the higher or tertier hospital, increase the hospital tariffs and health expenditures (Ham et al 2010, Babic et al 2015).

The casemix method uses a one-episode tariff, which is used beginning when the patient is hospitalized and covers services until the patient is discharged from hospital (Adams 2012). Implementing casemix with one-episode tariffs can reduce the rate of unnecessary admissions (Wadhwa and Duncan 2018).

### d. Billing and payment

The FFS method required a billing slip (Green & Rowell 2016). The need for more data and documents resulted in more time managing each bill in the billing process. The billing process for the casemix method does not require a service transaction receipt; instead, the total patient bill is determined from the coding results and the grouping of the patient data to generate the casemix charge (Adams 2012, Buck 2012). Casemix implementation reduced the number of documents for billing process (Buck 2012). The selection of payment method has an impact on cost reduction for services and on the costs of administration (Folland & Goodman 2014).

## 2.2.4 Casemix Implementation in Indonesia

In Indonesia, casemix was implemented in the national health security system in 2008. Before the implementation of casemix, activities were undertaken to prepare and calculate the casemix method that is used in Indonesia today. The preparations began in 2006, and the system was gradually implemented in 2008 in 15 vertical hospitals.

Table 2.4 History of casemix in Indonesia

| Year | Activities |
| --- | --- |
| 2006–2007 | Preparation and data collection |
| July 2007 | INA-DRG and charge system |
| July–August 2007 | Test the INA-DRG charge and grouping application |
| Sept 1, 2007 | Launch of the INA-DRG by the MOH |
| Sept 2007–Sept 2008 | Education and training for the INA-DRG system |
| Sept 1, 2008 | Casemix implementation in 15 vertical hospitals |
| Jan 1, 2009 | Casemix implementation in province and regional hospitals |
| 2011 | Revision of casemix charge |
| January 2013 | Launch of the INA-CBG revision 2012 |
| 2013 | Preparation for UHC—Jaminan Kesehatan Nasional (JKN) |
| January 2014 | Implementation of the INA-CBGs for UHC (the JKN programme) |
| December 2017 | 5,958 hospitals use the casemix method under Indonesia's UHC programme managed by BPJS |

Source: MOH 2008, 2011, 2012, 2014, 2017

In Indonesia, the number of CBGs increased from 604 codes for inpatients and 135 codes for outpatients in 2008 to 635 codes for inpatients and 198 codes for outpatients in 2012, and in 2013 (in preparation for UHC), there were 635 codes for inpatients and 268 codes for outpatients. Increasing the amount of data collected can increase the number of CBGs (MOH 2016). Indonesia CBG (INA-CBG) codes consist of 4 parts (MOH 2015).

Table 2.5 Development of INA-CBGs from 2008 to 2013 in preparation of Indonesia universal health coverage

|  | INA- DRG (2008) | INA-CBG (2012) | INA-CBG for UHC (2013) |
|---|---|---|---|
| Number of records coded | 127,354 | 1,048,475 | 6,000,000 |
| Sources of cost data | 13 hospitals | 100 hospitals | 137 hospitals |
| Period of data collection | 2006 | 2010 | 2011 |
| Contributors of cost data | Hospital type A and B | Hospital type A, B, C, and D and special hospitals | All types of hospitals and private hospitals |
| Number of CBGs | 739 (IPD 604, OPD 135) | 833 (IPD 635, OPD 198) | 903 (IPD 635, OPD 268) |
| Number of INA-CBGs | 1077 | 1077 | 1077 + 6 special CMG |
| Regional charge | - | 4 regional areas | 4 regional areas |
| Ward charge | Ward class 3 | Ward class 3 | Ward class 3,2,1 |

Source: MOH 2008, 2012, 2013.

As an archipelago country, Indonesia has a very large number of islands (16,056) and different economic conditions among regions. Typically, the eastern regions have higher transportation costs and more expensive prices than the western regions. INA-CBGs have adopted regionalisation charges to address these different conditions in the four regions:

1. Region 1 includes Java and Bali.
2. Region 2 includes Sumatera.
3. Region 3 includes Borneo (Kalimantan), Celebes (Sulawesi), and West Nusa Tenggara.
4. Region 4 includes East Nusa Tenggara, Maluku and Papua

The four regional charges indicate the additional charge associated with the region's location within the archipelago country. The additional charge consists of additional transportation and extra costs. Region 1 has the cheapest charge, and regions 2, 3 and 4 are progressively more expensive. Region 4 is the farthest region and has the most expensive charges (MOH 2016).

The INA-CBGs use 4-part codes consisting of the following (Aljunid 2012, MOH 2016):

1.  Casemix main group (CMG),
2.  Case type,
3.  CBG number, and
4.  Resource intensity/Severity level.

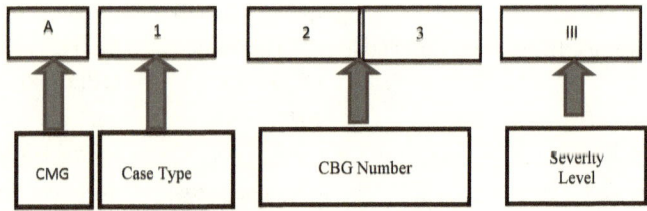

Figure 2.4 Indonesian case-base group (INA-CBG) codes
Source: The Indonesia Case-Base Groups (INA-CBG's) Tariff. The Ministry of Health. 2016

The first digit of the code represents the CMG. Thirty-two CMGs are used in the INA-CBGs for outpatient and inpatient services (MOH 2016):

Table 2.6 Casemix main group (CMG) codes used in the INA-CBGs

| No | Description | CMG Codes |
|----|-------------|-----------|
| 1 | Central nervous system groups | G |
| 2 | Eye and adnexa groups | H |
| 3 | Ear, nose, mouth & throat groups | U |
| 4 | Respiratory system groups | J |
| 5 | Cardiovascular system groups | I |
| 6 | Digestive system groups | K |
| 7 | Hepatobiliary & pancreatic system groups | B |
| 8 | Musculoskeletal system & connective tissue groups | M |
| 9 | Skin, subcutaneous tissue & breast groups | L |
| 10 | Endocrine system, nutrition & metabolism groups | E |
| 11 | Nephron-urinary system groups | N |
| 12 | Male reproductive system groups | V |
| 13 | Female reproductive system groups | W |
| 14 | Deliveries groups | O |
| 15 | Newborns and neonates groups | P |
| 16 | Haematopoietic & immune system groups | D |
| 17 | Myeloproliferative system & neoplasms groups | C |
| 18 | Infectious & parasitic diseases groups | A |
| 19 | Mental health &behavioural groups | F |
| 20 | Substance abuse & dependence groups | T |
| 21 | Injuries, poisonings & toxic effects of drugs groups | S |
| 22 | Factors influencing health status & other contacts with health services groups | Z |
| 23 | Ambulatory group—episodic | Q |
| 24 | Ambulatory group—package | QP |
| 25 | Sub-acute groups | SA |
| 26 | Special procedures | YY |
| 27 | Special drugs | DD |
| 28 | Special investigations I | II |
| 29 | Special investigations II | IJ |
| 30 | Special prothesis | RR |
| 31 | Chronic groups | CD |
| 32 | Error CMGs | X |

Source: The Central of Financing Health Insurance (MOH 2014)

The second digit of the code represents the type of case according to the INA-CBG code. These codes describe the types of cases that are served by hospitals and are listed below (MOH 2016):

1. Outpatient without procedure
2. Outpatient with minor procedure
3. Outpatient with major procedure
4. Inpatient without procedure
5. Inpatient with minor procedure
6. Inpatient with major procedure
7. Outpatient neonatal
8. Inpatient neonatal
9. Error

The third and fourth digits of the code describe the case base for the CMG and have gradually been improved in the casemix system. There were 759 CBGs in 2008, 833 CBGs in 2012 and 851 CBGs in 2013. The fifth digit of the code indicates the severity level of the case, and there are 3 codes for severity level:

    a. Code I   : without complication
    b. Code II  : with minor complication
    c. Code III : with major complication

In Indonesia, the casemix method for hospital reimbursement has been implemented using INA-CBGs based on UNU-Grouper. The casemix method represents one episode of patient treatment consisting of doctor consultations, medical procedures, diagnostic procedures, drugs, wards, etc. and is based on clinical pathways that provide clinical practice guidelines for medical care. Typically, for inpatient care, one episode starts with admission and ends when the patient is discharged (MOH 2014, MOH 2016).

In Indonesia, the billing process for casemix does not require all of a patient's bills to make a claim for the patient. All the data in the complete medical chart are processed and grouped by the INA-CBG Grouper software; these data then become a patient's claim and can be printed to become part of a patient claim's documentation (MOH 2011, 2014, 2016).

The hospital information system is integrated with the INA-CBG Grouper software and the patient registration software. When a patient is discharged, medical records or medical charts are coded using ICD-10 and ICD-9-CM and grouped by the INA-CBG Grouper software, which determines the INA-CBG code and charge. The hospital sends a softcopy of the patients' claim and the summary claim report to the payer every month. The payer verifies the claim documents and determines whether or not the claims are approved for payment. If the documents are not approved, the payer informs the hospital of the need to revise or complete the unapproved claim documents. If the claim documents are verified and approved, the payer pays the hospital's claim based on the verification result.

The hospital must prepare the following claim documents as attachments to a claim (MOH 2011):

1. Copy of Jamkesmas card
2. Referral letter from the lower-level hospital
3. Copy of Indonesia Family Card
4. National Identity Card

    a. Copy of Indonesia National Identity Card for adult patients (17 years old and older)
    b. Copy of Indonesia National Identity Card for the parents of paediatric patients

5. Letter of Health Service Insurance (Surat Jaminan Pelayanan=SJP)
6. Medical chart with ICD-10 and ICD-9-CM codes
7. The results from the INA-CBG Grouper software
8. Certain bills only for thalassemia drugs, haemophilia drugs, and cardiac and orthopaedic stent

9. The total of one patient's bill (inpatients only)
10. Doctor's instructions for discharged patients
11. Death certificate (for patients who died in the hospitals

All the prepared documents consist of original documents. To deliver a claim to the payer, the hospital must also prepare a cover letter with the total hospital claim and approval from the Hospital Medical Committee for cases at the 3rd level of severity and then send an email to the payer with all of the hospital's claim documents as attachments. The payer verifies and pays the hospital claim, or the payer rejects the claim and sends it back for revision or for completion of the claim documents (MOH 2011, 2016).

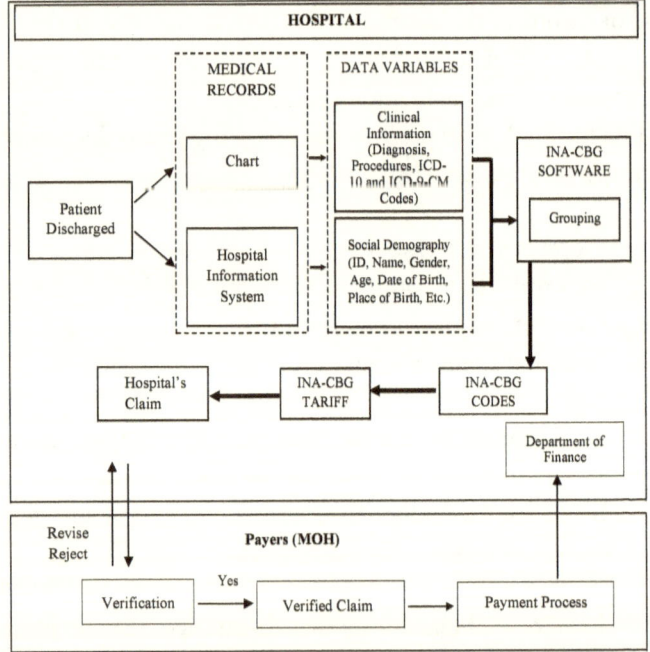

Figure 2.5 Billing process for the casemix payment method
Source: The Guidelines of Jaminan Kesehatan
Masyarakat Programme. MOH 2011;Guide to Medical
Billing and Coding (ICDC 2007); Delivery
Source: MOH 2011,2016; Adams (2012).

## 2.3 Flowchart of Study Activities

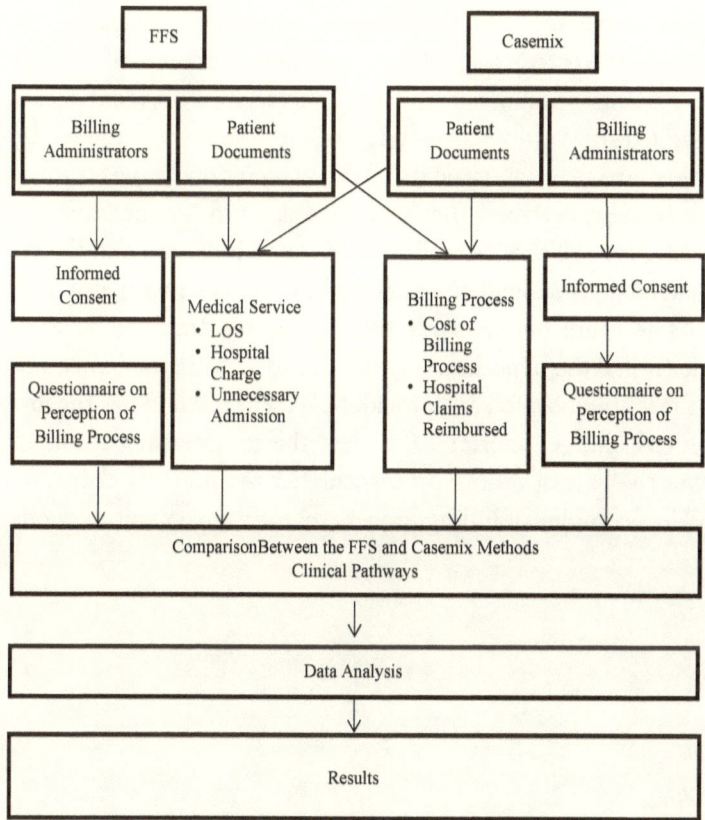

Figure 2.6 Flowchart of study activities

To fulfil the research objectives, this flowchart of study activities collected 2 groups of patient documents in the medical services and the billing process that used the FFS and casemix payment method as tariff reimbursement. From both groups of patients data, we studied the variables of LOS, hospital charge and unnecesary admission in the medical service; cost of billing process and hospital claims paid in the billing process. Also, the study surveyed the perception of billing administrators using the questionnaire for describing the billing process that used the FFS and casemix payment method.

All data of both group payment methods (FFS and casemix) were analysed by descriptive. Length of stay, hospital charge, unnecessary admission, the cost of billing process, hospital claims paid and the perception of billing process were compared between the patients reimbursed by FFS and casemix payment method using t-test. Multiple logistic regression was used in the medical service analysis for evaluating the association between all the independent variables (hospital charge, LOS, gender, age, type of case, type of service, and unnecessary admission) and the type of payment as dependent variable (FFS =0; casemix method =1).

The result of this study fulfiled the research objectives and determined the hypotheses wheather the casemix implementation in a teaching hospital as a provider payment method has the lower hospital charge, shorter LOS, less the unnecessary admission, lower the cost of billing process, higher the hospital claims paid and less complex of billing process than FFS payment method.

 METHODOLOGY

## 3.1  Study Design

This is a cross-sectional study using retrospective data to compare the impact of the casemix and FFS reimbursement methods (Notoatmojo 2010, Widi 2010).

## 3.2  Study Site

The Cipto Mangunkusumo Central National Referral Hospital (RSCM) is a government-owned referral and teaching hospital located in central Jakarta. RSCM is the largest hospital in Indonesia with 1,001 public beds and 74 private beds in its International Wing. The average length of stay (ALOS) is 5.5 days, and the bed-occupancy rate (BOR) is 80.0%. The average number of outpatient visits per day is 4,075. As the largest national hospital in Indonesia, the hospital has 5,089 employees consisting of 6 directors, 601 doctors, 1,946 nurses, 787 medical support employees, 1,755 administrators, and 2,430 medical students (RSCM 2017).

RSCM has 24 medical departments and 167 medical divisions in several medical buildings, namely, building "A" (public wards building), the Kencana building for International and VVIP-class patients, the Cardiac Centre building, the Emergency building, the Central Integrated Surgery building with Intensive Care Unit and Intensive Care Cardiac Unit, the Central Medical Unit building I-III, the Geriatric building, the Psychiatric building, the Kiara building (mother and child care centre), the Kirana building (eye centre), the Kintani building (women's health centre for outpatient services), the Dental Care Centre building, the Radiotherapy building, the Radiology building, the Medical Rehabilitation building, the Outpatient building, the Forensic building, the Administration building, the Medical Staff building, and public service facilities. The medical expertise provided by sub-specialized medical doctors and excellent facilities are available at RSCM for all patients. RSCM was accredited by the Ministry of Health (MOH) and the Joint Commission International (JCI) in 2013 and 2016 (RSCM 2017).

To support national and regional health insurance programmes, RSCM employed two different reimbursement methods for patients covered by different social health insurance programmes. FFS was used for the Gakin (Keluarga Maskin, or poor families) programme run by the Jakarta provincial government, and casemix was used for the Jaminan Kesehatan Masyarakat (Jamkesmas, public health insurance) programme of the Indonesian MOH (RSCM 2012). Currently, RSCM provides health care services for Indonesia's universal health coverage (UHC) programme.

## 3.3  Study Duration

This study was conducted over a span of four years.

## 3.4    Study Activities

To fulfil the objectives of the study, the study activities were divided into 3 sub-studies as follows:

1. Review of the hospital's annual reports
2. Review of medical services

    a. Review of patients' medical records for the five most common primary diagnoses for inpatients and outpatients
    b. Review of unnecessary admissions

3. Review of billing process

    a. Review of the cost of the billing process
    b. Review of the hospital's claims reimbursed
    c. Survey of perceptions of the billing process

### 3.4.1  Review of The Hospital's Annual Reports

This section fulfils the research objective to describe the social demography and classification of the primary diagnoses of patients whose costs were reimbursed using the casemix system under the social health insurance scheme.

### a.  Sampling frame

The sampling frame of this study consisted of the list of patients insured under the Gakin programme using the FFS payment method and the list of patients insured under the Jamkesmas programme using the casemix payment method. The data were sourced from January 1$^{st}$ to December 31$^{st}$ 2011 for inpatient services and from January 1$^{st}$ to March 31$^{st}$ 2011 for outpatient services.

## b. Inclusion and exclusion criteria

### i) Inclusion criteria

1. All inpatients discharged during the period from January 1st to December 31st 2011
2. All outpatients who visited the hospital during the period from January 1st to March 31st 2011
3. All patients covered under the Gakin and Jamkesmas programmes

### ii) Exclusion criteria

1. All patients covered by other health insurance programmes
2. All patients who paid for their own health services
3. All inpatients discharged from inpatient services before or after the period from January 1st to December 31st 2011
4. All outpatients who visited outpatient services before or after the period from January 1st to March 31st 2011

## c. Sampling method

The universal sampling method was used to capture all patients who fulfilled the inclusion and exclusion criteria. The inpatient samples comprised all patients in public wards (3rd-class wards) during the period from January 1st to December 31st 2011 for inpatient services and from January 1st to March 31st 2011 for outpatient services under the Jamkesmas and Gakin programmes.

## d. Source of data

This study used data obtained from the monthly patient reports for the Jamkesmas and Gakin programmes in 2011.

## e. Study tools

The study tools included the International Classification of Diseases, Tenth Revision (ICD-10, WHO 2008), electronic health records (EHRs) from the hospital management information system (HMIS) and SPSS version 22.

## f. Data collection

Most of patient data under Gakin programme that reimbursed by the FFS method was documented manually in hard copy and only several data were documented in excel file. In 2011, there were not computerized integratedly for all data of patient admission, services and billing. Those data were collected manually one by one during data collection periode. The collecting data started from the hospital claim report in the Financial Departement, then were added data of age and gender from the patient admission in the Patient Insurance Services Unit (UPPJ). The next step, the primary diagnoses were coded by ICD 10. If the primary diagnoses were not available in the hospital claim report, the researcher looked for the information from the Medical Record Unit. The data collection for the patient using the FFS needed longer time than the casemix method.

Patients under Jamkesmas programme used the INA-CBG's software in th Patient Insurance Services Unit (UPPJ), but many data of patient demography were blank. The researcher completed data manually from the patient medical records or the patient admission. Mostly, the data of patients under Jamkesmas reimbursed by the casemix were more complete than the FFS method.

Data on patients' gender, age, referral area and primary diagnosis were grouped to the data of FFS method and the data of casemix method.

## g. Data analysis

The data on gender, age, referral area and primary diagnosis were trimmed by 5% (Lwanga and Lemeshow 1991) then analysed by the descriptive method and reported in tabulations using SPSS version 22.

## 3.4.2 Review of Medical Records

The review is divided into 2 sub-studies:

1. review of patients' medical records for the five most common diagnoses, and
2. review of unnecessary admissions.

## a. Review of patients' medical records for the five most common diagnoses

This section fulfils the research objective to determine and compare hospital charge and length of stay (LOS) for patients whose costs were reimbursed through the casemix and FFS methods.

### i) Sampling frame

The sampling frame of this sub-study was the list of patients with the five most common diagnoses under the Gakin programme using the FFS method and under the Jamkesmas programme using the casemix method during the period from January 1st to December 31st 2011 for inpatient services and during the period from January 1st to March 31st 2011 for outpatient services.

## ii) Inclusion and exclusion criteria

### Inclusion criteria

1.  Patients on the list who had one of the five most common diagnoses who were under the Gakin programme and whose costs were reimbursed using the FFS payment method for outpatient and inpatient services and patients on the list who had one of the five most common diagnosis who were under the Jamkesmas programme and whose costs were reimbursed using the casemix system for outpatient and inpatient services.
2.  Outpatients who visited from January 1$^{st}$ to March 31$^{st}$ 2011 and inpatients discharged from January 1$^{st}$ to December 31$^{st}$ 2011.

### Exclusion criteria

1.  Patients on the list who did not have one of the five most common diagnoses.
2.  Patients not covered by the Gakin or Jamkesmas programmes.
3.  Outpatients who visited outside of the period from January 1$^{st}$ to March 31$^{st}$ 2011 and all inpatients who were discharged outside the period from January 1$^{st}$ to December 31$^{st}$ 2011.

## iii) Sampling methods

Universal sampling was used in this study. The samples were patients with one the five most common diagnoses for outpatient services from January 1$^{st}$ to March 31$^{st}$ and for inpatient services during the period from January 1$^{st}$ to December 31$^{st}$ 2011 who were under the Gakin programme using the FFS method or under the Jamkesmas programme using the casemix method.

## iv) Estimation of sample size

The Lemeshow formula was used to estimate the sample size for this sub-study with 95% confidence intervals and 90% power (Hosmer and Lemeshow 1989, Pandey 1999). The results of research research on the system-wide impacts of hospital payment reforms in Central and Eastern Europe and Central Asia (Moreno-Serra and Wagstaff 2009) were used in this calculation: the mean for LOS in public hospitals was 11.55 (SD 2.13) for the FFS payment method and 10.73 (SD 2.01) for the casemix payment method.

$$n = \frac{2\sigma^2 \left| Z_{1-\alpha/2} + Z_{1-\beta} \right|^2}{(\mu_1 - \mu_2)^2}$$

$$n = \frac{\frac{2\,(2.13^2 + 2.01^2)}{2} \times (1.96 + 1.282)^2}{(11.55 - 10.73)^2}$$

$$n = \frac{(4.54 + 4.04) \times (10.51)}{0.82^2}$$

$$n = \frac{8.58 \times 10.51}{0.67}$$

$$n = 134.59 \approx 135$$

n        = number of samples

$\sigma^2$        = pooled standard deviation is $(\sigma_1^2 + \sigma_2^2)/2$

$Z_{1-\alpha/2}$  = 1.96 for 95% confidence interval

$Z_{1-\beta}$     = 1.282 for 90% power

$\mu_1$      = mean of LOS under the FFS payment method

$\mu_2$      = mean of LOS under the casemix payment method

The estimated number of samples was 135 patients for each diagnosis group of the five most common diagnoses; and the total number of samples in the five most common diagnoses among patients whose costs were reimbursed under FFS and casemix was 675 patients respectively. The total number of inpatients and outpatients whose costs were reimbursed by casemix was 1,350 samples, which was similar to the total number of samples for patients reimbursed under FFS. There were 2,700 total samples for this sub-study.

### v) Source of data

The data sources used in this study were as follows:

— medical records for patients under the FFS (Gakin) and casemix (Jamkesmas) methods who were diagnosed with one of the five most common diagnoses from January 1st to December 31st 2011 for inpatient services and from January 1st 2011 to March 31st 2011 for outpatient services, and

— patient billing reports for patients under the FFS (Gakin) and casemix (Jamkesmas) methods who were diagnosed with one of the five most common diagnoses for outpatient and inpatient services in 2011.

### vi) Study tools

The tools used in this study included the following:

— the ICD-10 (WHO 2008),
— the International Classification of Diseases, Ninth Revision, Clinical Modification (WHO 2008),
— the Grouper software for Indonesian case-base groups (INA-CBG) version 3.2 based on United Nations University (UNU)-Grouper (MOH 2011),
— EHRs from the HMIS, and
— SPSS version 22.

## vii) Data collection

The sample data of the hospital's annual reports were completed by the secondary/ tertiary diagnoses and procedures from the patient medical records in the Medical Records Unit. For the patients reimbursed by the casemix method, the diagnoses and the procedures were available in the INA-CBG's software.

Contrarily, all the sample data of patients under the FFS method were completed manually with secondary/tertiary diagnoses and procedures from the patient medical records, then were coded by the ICD-10 for diagnoses and ICD-9-CM for procedures. All of data were grouped using the INA-CBG Grouper software version 3.2. With the huge number of patients reimbursed by the FFS method, these processes were the longest period in this study. Finding the patient medical records during 2 or 3 years ago were not easy in that time, and the limited coders and budget also become the challenges in this data collection.

After both the group of patient data were already completed, those data were sorted by the frequency. The five most common diagnoses were obtained from the records of patients under the FFS method, and the same diagnoses were obtained from the documents of patients under the casemix method.

## viii) Data analysis

The five most common diagnoses in both groups of patients were analysed by descriptive statistics, and normality was evaluated using the Kolmogorov-Smirnov test. The comparisons between FFS and casemix patients for hospital charge and LOS were analysed by t-tests using SPSS version 22 with 95% confidence levels (Pett 2016, Gerstman 2015, Dahlan 2009).

## ix) Variables

Table 3.1 The dependent and independent variables in the review of
medical records for the five most common diagnoses

| No | Variables | Definition of Term |
|----|-----------|--------------------|
| 1 | Dependent: Type of Payment | |
| | Fee-for-service | Fee-for-service (FFS) is retrospective payment to a provider for each act or service rendered (WHO 2001). |
| | Casemix | Casemix is a classification of patient treatment episodes designed to create classes that are relatively homogenous with respect the resources used and that contain patients with similar clinical characteristics (Green et al 2016). |
| 2 | Independent | |
| | Hospital tariff | Hospital tariff was the payment received by hospitals on the medical service or non-medical service that were done to the patients (MOH 2015) |
| | Length of stay | Length of stay (LOS) is the period of time a patient remains in a hospital or other health care facility as an inpatient (WHO 2001). |

For this sub study, the variables were used as below:

## b. Review of unnecessary admission cases

This section fulfils the research objective to compare the
rates of unnecessary admissions for patients whose costs were
reimbursed using the casemix and FFS methods.

## i) Sampling frame

The sampling frame for this sub-study was the list of Gakin
patients whose costs were reimbursed through FFS and Jamkesmas
patients whose costs were reimbursed through casemix who were
admitted for one day to the emergency unit or public wards and

were discharged in better condition and were not referred out to other facilities from January 1$^{st}$ to December 31$^{st}$ 2011.

## ii) Inclusion and exclusion criteria

### Inclusion criteria

1. Patients in the Jamkesmas programme whose costs were reimbursed using the casemix method and who had a one-day LOS in the emergency unit or a public ward and who were discharged in better condition and who were not referred out to other facilities from January 1$^{st}$ to December 31$^{st}$ 2011.
2. Patients in the Gakin programme whose costs were reimbursed using the FFS method and who had a one-day LOS in the emergency unit or a public ward and who were discharged in better condition and who were not referred out to other facilities from January 1$^{st}$ to December 31$^{st}$ 2011.

### Exclusion criteria

1. Patients in the Jamkesmas and Gakin programmes with an LOS of more than one day.
2. Cases covered by other health insurance programmes.
3. Patients who paid for their health services at their own expense.
4. Patients who stayed for one day or less but died on the first day of admission.
5. Patients who stayed for one day or less but were referred out to the other hospitals.
6. Patients who stayed for one day or less outside the period from January 1$^{st}$ to December 31$^{st}$ 2011.

### iii) Sampling method

The List of Emergency Diagnosis that are covered by the National Health Security System. There were 189 diagnoses consisted of 31 for pediatric, 68 for surgery, 17 for cardiovascular, 12 for obstetrics and gynecology,12 for eye, 15 for pulmonology, 17 for internal diseases, 13 for ear, nose and throat, 4 for psychiatry. All these diagnoses were covered by the social health insurance, and patients with these diagnoses were categorized as necessary admission through emergency unit (MOH 2014).

The sample for unnecessary admissions was defined as patients who were hospitalized through the emergency unit, had a one-day hospitalization in the emergency unit or the third-class ward (public ward), were discharged from the hospital in better condition, were not referred out to other health care facilities, and had a diagnosis that was not listed in emergency diagnosis list in Indonesia's MOH Regulation Number 903/Menkes/PER/V/2011 (MOH 2011). The sample was selected by the universal sampling method, and patients who met the definition were included in the sample for this sub-study.

### iv) Estimation of sample size

The estimation of sample size used the formula for the difference between two proportions for an analytical study with a risk difference of 5 percentage points and a 95% confidence interval (Lwanga and Lemeshow1991). The research findings of the National DRG Validation Study: Unnecessary Admissions to Hospitals (Kusserow 1988) were used in this calculation: a 12.5 percent rate of unnecessary admission for non-teaching hospitals and an 8.8 percent rate for teaching hospitals.

$$V=P_1 (1-P_1) + P_2(1-P_2)$$
$$V=0.125(1-0.125) + 0.088(1-0.088)$$
$$V=(0.125*0.875) + 0.088(0.912)$$
$$V=0.109 + 0.080$$
$$V= 0.189 \approx 0.19$$

$V$ = Intermediate value

$P_1$ = Population proportion of the FFS payment method

$P_2$ = Population proportion of the casemix payment method

$d$  = Absolute precision 5% in confidence level 95%

According to the calculation, the Vvalue was 0.19. With 5 percentage points of the absolute precision ($d$) and a Vvalue of 0.19, the number of samples were determined from the table of sample size for confidence level 96% (Lwanga and Lemeshow 1991).

Table 3.2 The sampling size of unnecessary admission for confidence level 95 %

| $d$ / $V$ | 0.01 | 0.02 | 0.03 | 0.04 | 0.05 |
|---|---|---|---|---|---|
| 0.01 | 385 | 97 | 43 | 25 | 16 |
| 0.02 | 769 | 193 | 86 | 49 | 31 |
| 0.03 | 1153 | 289 | 129 | 73 | 47 |
| 0.04 | 1537 | 385 | 171 | 97 | 62 |
| 0.05 | 1921 | 481 | 214 | 121 | 77 |
| 0.06 | 2306 | 577 | 257 | 145 | 93 |
| 0.07 | 2690 | 673 | 299 | 169 | 108 |
| 0.08 | 3074 | 768 | 342 | 193 | 123 |
| 0.09 | 3458 | 865 | 385 | 217 | 139 |
| 0.10 | 3842 | 961 | 427 | 241 | 154 |
| 0.12 | 4610 | 1153 | 513 | 289 | 185 |
| 0.14 | 5379 | 1345 | 598 | 337 | 216 |
| 0.16 | 6147 | 1537 | 683 | 385 | 246 |
| 0.18 | 6915 | 1729 | 769 | 433 | 277 |
| 0.20 | 7684 | 1921 | 854 | 481 | 308 |
| 0.22 | 8452 | 2113 | 940 | 529 | 339 |
| 0.24 | 9220 | 2305 | 1025 | 577 | 369 |

0.19 ➡ (row 0.20) ⬅ 292.5

Source : Sample size determination in health students – A practical Manual. Lwanga and Lemeshow 1991

From the table of sample size above, Vvalue of 0.19 was between Vvalue of 0.18 for 272 samples and Vvalue of 0.20 for 308 samples. Vvalue of 0.19 was (272+308)/2= 292.5≈ 293. The estimated number of samples was 293 for each reimbursement method group. To address the issue of incomplete information in the patients' medical records, 300 cases were selected from each group (FFS and casemix payment methods).

## v) Source of data

The data sources used in this study were as follows:

— the medical records of patients with a one-day LOS whose costs were reimbursed under the FFS method (Gakin) and the casemix method (Jamkesmas) from January 1st to December 31st 2011.
— the billing reports for patients with a one-day LOS whose costs were reimbursed under the FFS method (Gakin) and the casemix method (Jamkesmas, Jampersal, and Jampelthas) during the period from January 1st to December 31st 2011.

## vi) Study tools

The following tools were used in this study:

1. MOH Regulation Number 903/Menkes/PER/V/2011,
2. EHRs from the HMIS,
3. the INA-CBG Grouper software version 3.2 based on UNU-Grouper (MOH 2011),
4. the ICD-10,
5. the ICD-9 CM, and
6. SPSS version 22.

## vii) Data collection

The sample data of the hospital's annual reports of the FFS and the casemix method were completed by length of stay from the emergency unit and the Patient Insurance Services Unit (UPPJ). Those data were collected by one-day hospitalizations (LOS=1) as the data of necessary and unnecessary admission. Then, the LOS=1-group data were completed with referral letter from UPPJ and hospital charges from the Financial Department. Also, the researcher completed with the primary diagnoses from the data of the review of patients' medical records for the five most common primary diagnoses (see 3.4.2.a.vii page 49).

Then, the both of LOS=1-group data were selected by using the emergency diagnosis list of Indonesian MOH Regulation Number 903/Menkes/PER/V/2011. Patients with a diagnosis that was not in the emergency diagnosis list of the Indonesian Ministry of Health Regulation Number 903/Menkes/PER/V/2011 were categorized as unnecessary admission samples. And the rest of samples that were not catagorized as unnecessary admission became as necessary admission.

During the collection data, there were not available the hospital integrated information system. All processes of these data selection were done manually in the emergency unit for data LOS=1, in UPPJ for referral letter, in the Financial Department for hospital charges, then, were completed with the primary diagnoses.

## viii) Data analysis

The proportion of unnecessary admissions and the proportion of referral letter usage for patients under the FFS and casemix methods were compared using the Chi-square test with SPSS version 22 and 95% confidence levels (Pett 2016, Walker 2011, Dahlan 2009).

## ix) Variables

This sub study used the variables as below:

Table 3.3 The dependent and independent variables in the review of unnecessary admission cases

| No | Variables | Definition of Term |
|----|-----------|---------------------|
| 1 | Dependent: Type of Payment | |
| | Fee-for-service | Fee-for-service (FFS) is retrospective payment to a provider for each act or service rendered (WHO 2001). |
| | Casemix | Casemix is a classification of patient treatment episodes designed to create classes that are relatively homogenous with respect the resources used and that contain patients with similar clinical characteristics (Green et al 2016). |
| 2 | Independent Unnecessary admission | Unnecessary admission consist of a person who is admitted to a hospital as an inpatient and spends one day or less in the hospital, even though his/her condition did not warrant admission (Miller 2003). |

## c Regression analysis for medical records review

Multiple regression analysis was used to evaluate the association between all the independent variables and the dependent variable: type of payment (FFS or casemix method). Based on the 2 sub-studies above (review of patients' medical records for the five most common diagnoses and review of unnecessary admissions), the researcher collected and trimmed 5% of the data (Lwanga 1991, Pett 2016). The dependent variable was type of payment, i.e., FFS or casemix, and the independent variables were hospital charge, LOS, gender, age, type of case, type of service, and unnecessary admission. A correlation test was conducted to determine the strength of the relationship between variables by using Spearman's test (Pett 2016, Gerstman 2015).

A regression analysis was performed to study the dependent variable and one or more independent variables (Pett 2016, Gerstman 2015). Binary logistic regression analysis was selected; the dependent variable, type of payment, was categorized as FFS method=0 and casemix method=1, and the independent variables were LOS, hospital charge, gender (male=0; female=1), age, type of case (medical=0; surgical=1), type of service (outpatient=0; inpatient=1), and unnecessary admission (necessary admission=0; unnecessary admission=1).

The hypotheses for the logistic regression model were as follows:

- $H_o$: The independent variables LOS, hospital charge, gender, age, type of case, type of service, and unnecessary admission are not associated with the dependent variable, type of payment (FFS or casemix method).
- $H_1$: The independent variables LOS, hospital charge, gender, age, type of case, type of service, and unnecessary admission are associated with the dependent variable, type of payment (FFS or casemix method).

The omnibus value test was used to analyse the validity of the regression model. Meanwhile, Nagelkerke's R-square was used to determine the goodness of fit of the logistic regression model using SPSS software with 95% confidence levels (Pett 2016, Gerstmann 2015, Dahlan 2009).

Table 3.4 The dependent and independent variables in the multiple
logistic regression analysis of the review of medical services

| No | Variables | Definition of Term |
|---|---|---|
| 1 | Dependent: Type of Payment | |
| | Fee-for-service | Fee-for-service (FFS) is retrospective payment to a provider for each act or service rendered (WHO 2001). |
| | Casemix | Casemix is a classification of patient treatment episodes designed to create classes that are relatively homogenous with respect the resources used and that contain patients with similar clinical characteristics (Green et al 2016). |
| 2 | Independent | |
| | Hospital tariff | Hospital tariff was the payment received by hospitals on the medical service or non-medical service that were done to the patients (MOH 2015) |
| | Length of stay | Length of stay (LOS) is the period of time a patient remains in a hospital or other health care facility as an inpatient (Cashin 2015). |
| | Type of cases | Type of cases determined whether cases with surgical procedures (surgical cases) or withour surgical cases (medical cases) (MOH 2016) |
| | Type of services | Type of services determined whether patients had the health service in outpatient or inpatient services |
| | Gender | Gender of patient |
| | Age | Age of patient in years |
| | Unnecessary admission | An unnecessary admission consists of a person who is admitted to a hospital as an inpatient and spends one day or less in the hospital, even though his/her condition did not warrant admission (Means 2016). |

### 3.4.3 Review of Billing Process

This review fulfils the objectives of the study via 3 activities:

1.  Review of the cost of the billing process,
2.  Review of the percentage of hospital claims paid, and
3.  Survey of perceptions of the billing process.

### a. Review of the costs of the billing process

This study fulfils the research objective to analyse the costs of the billing process for patients reimbursed using the casemix and FFS methods.

### i) Sampling frame

The sampling frame was a list of the costs of the billing process from hospital financial reports for patients in the Gakin and Jamkesmas programmes who received inpatient and outpatient services during the period from January 1$^{st}$ to December 31$^{st}$ 2011.

The costs of the billing process include the costs required to prepare patients' bills through hospital claim delivery. Indirect costs were not included in the calculated costs, while direct costs, which showed clear separation between the FFS and casemix billing costs, served as the data in this sub-study. The bill preparation costs consisted of fees associated with employees, such as salary, incentives, overtime pay, and the employee meal allowance as well as transport fees and costs for office stationery, photocopies and software maintenance.

### ii) Inclusion and exclusion criteria

### Inclusion criteria

1.  The costs of the billing process for patients in the Gakin and Jamkesmas programmes during the period from January 1$^{st}$ to December 31$^{st}$ 2011.

2. The costs of the billing process related to human resources, transportation and stationery from the hospital financial reports for 2011.

**Exclusion criteria**

1. The costs of the billing process for patients other than those in the Gakin and Jamkesmas programmes during the period from January 1st to December 31st 2011.
2. The costs of the billing process other than those related to human resources, stationery and transportation.

### iii) Sampling method

The universal sampling method was used to collect human resources costs, stationery costs and transportation costs related to the billing process for the Gakin programme and the Jamkesmas programme during the period from January 1st to December 31st 2011 from the 2011 hospital financial reports.

### iv) Source of data

The data sources for this study were the hospital's financial reports from 2011 and the hospital's claim reports from 2011 and 2012.

### v) Study tools

The tools used in this sub-study were the Technical Guidelines of the 2011 Gakin programme (PHOJP 2011), the 2011 Guidelines of the Jaminan Kesehatan Masyarakat Programme (MOH 2011), and the EHR software.

### vi) Data collection

The cost of the billing process was collected from the financial department and from the 2011 hospital financial reports. The cost of the billing process excluded indirect costs and shared costs such as electricity, water, and telephone. In this study, the collected costs of the billing process were clearly separated between the FFS and casemix methods. The cost of the billing process consisted of the following:

— human resources costs: wages, renumeration, and overtime fees;
— stationery costs: office and computer equipment costs, photocopy costs, the cost of software maintenance;
— transportation costs: the cost of delivering claims to the payer, transportation cost for payer's verifiers.

The data were divided into two groups, namely, the cost of the billing process under the FFS method and the cost of the billing process under the casemix method. The number of patients per year was collected from the hospital claim report to calculate the cost of the billing process per patient.

## vii) Data analysis

The costs for human resources, transportation and stationery were calculated for each month during the year for both the FFS and casemix methods. Those data were analysed using Kolmogorov-Smirnov normality test. The costs of human resources, transportation, and stationery for the FFS and casemix methods were compared via t-tests using SPSS version 22 with 95% confidence levels (Pett 2016, Gerstman 2015, Dahlan 2009).

The cost of the billing process per patient was calculated by dividing the total cost of billing per year by the number of patients per year (Wenzel 2014).

$$\text{Cost of one patient's bill} = \frac{\text{total costs for one year}}{\text{number of patients in the year}}$$

$$\frac{\Delta \text{cost of}}{\text{1bill}} = \frac{(\text{cost of one patient's bill }_{FFS} - \text{cost of one patient's bill }_{casemix})}{\text{cost of one patient's bill }_{casemix}}$$

This calculation shows the cost of one patient's bill whose costs were reimbursed under the FFS method and the casemix method.

## ix) Variables

The variables that were used in this sub study as below:

Table 3.5 The dependent and independent variables in the review of the cost of billing proces

| No | Variables | Definition of Term |
|----|-----------|--------------------|
| 1 | Dependent : Type of Payment | |
| | Fee-for-service | Fee-for-service (FFS) is retrospective payment to a provider for each act or service rendered (WHO 2001). |
| | Casemix | Casemix is a classification of patient treatment episodes designed to create classes that are relatively homogenous with respect the resources used and that contain patients with similar clinical characteristics (Buck 2012). |
| 2 | Independent | |
| | The human resources cost | The human resources cost is the cost for employees such as wages, renumeration, overtimes fees, and insurance (RSCM 2017). |
| | The stationery cost | The stationery cost is the cost of paper, printer paper, computer ink, copies, computer maintenance, and containers for documents (RSCM 2017) |
| | The transportation cost | The transportation cost is the cost for delivering billing claims from the hospital to the payer's office and the cost of transportation for verifiers (RSCM 2017). |

## b. Review of Hospital Claims Reimbursed

This sub-study fulfils the research objective to compare the percentage of claims paid for patients whose costs were reimbursed using the casemix and FFS methods.

### i) Sampling frame

The sampling frame was the list of the hospital's claims paid under the Gakin and Jamkesmas programmes for inpatient and outpatient services during the period from January 1$^{st}$ to December 31$^{st}$ 2011.

### ii) Inclusion and exclusion criteria

### Inclusion criteria

Hospital claim payments for inpatients and outpatients under the Gakin and Jamkesmas programmes during the period from January 1$^{st}$ to December 31$^{st}$ 2011.

### Exclusion criteria

1.  Hospital claim payments that were not under the Gakin or Jamkesmas programmes.
2.  Hospital claim payments that were not generated during the period from January 1$^{st}$ to December 31$^{st}$ 2011.

### iii) Sampling method

The universal sampling method was used to obtain the list of the hospital's claim payments under the Gakin programme with FFS and the Jamkesmas programme with casemix for inpatient and outpatient services during the period from January 1$^{st}$ to December 31$^{st}$2011.

## iv) Source of data

The data source in this study was the Claim and Payment Reports in 2011 and 2012 for inpatient and outpatient services under the Gakin and Jamkesmas programmes.

## v) Study tools

The tools of this sub-study were EHRs from the HMIS, the 2011 Technical Guidelines for the Gakin programme (PHOJP 2011), and the 2011 Guidelines for the Jaminan Kesehatan Masyarakat (Jamkesmas) programme (MOH 2011).

## vi) Data collection

The data were collected in the financial department and the Patient Insurance Service Unit. The total hospital claims and the total claims paid per month for patients whose costs were reimbursed under the FFS method and the casemix method were collected for inpatients and outpatients during 2011 and 2012.

## vii) Data analysis

The percentage of each hospital claim paid was calculated for one year either for inpatient services or outpatient services as follows (Baker, 2004):

$$\% \text{ of claims paid } = \frac{\text{hospital claims paid by the payer}}{\text{hospital claims delivered by the hospital}} \times 100\%$$

The results for % of claims paid under the FFS and casemix methods were then compared using t-tests with 95% confidence levels.

## viii) Variables

In this sub study, the variabels were used as below:

Table 3.6 The dependent and independent variables in the review of
hospital claim reimbursed

| No | Variables | Definition of Term |
|---|---|---|
| 1 | Dependent : Type of Payment | |
| | Fee-for-service | Fee-for-service (FFS) is retrospective payment to a provider for each act or service rendered (WHO 2001). |
| | Casemix | Casemix is a classification of patient treatment episodes designed to create classes that are relatively homogenous with respect the resources used and that contain patients with similar clinical characteristics (Green et al 2016). |
| 2 | Independent | |
| | Hospital claim reimbursed | The hospital claim reimbursed is the payment of the hospital claims that are verified and approved by the payers (MOH 2018) |

## c. Survey on Perceptions of The Billing Process

This sub-study addressed the study objective to compare the
billing processes for the casemix and FFS methods.

## i) Sampling frame

The sampling frame for this sub-study included the billing
administrators in the financial department and the Patient
Insurance Service Unit who were involved directly in the billing
process for patients under the Gakin programme using FFS and
the Jamkesmas programme using casemix during the period from
January 1st to December 31st 2011.

## ii) Inclusion and exclusion criteria

### Inclusion criteria

Billing administrators in the financial department and the Patient Insurance Service Unit involved in the billing processes for the Gakin and Jamkesmas programmes during 2011.

### Exclusion criteria

Billing administrators who were never involved in the billing processes for patients in the Gakin and Jamkesmas programmes during the period from January 1st to December 31st 2011.

## iii) Sampling method

Universal sampling was used in this study to select billing administrators in the financial department and the Patient Insurance Service Unit according to their jobs and responsibilities related to the billing process for patients whose costs were reimbursed through FFS (Gakin programme) and casemix (Jamkesmas programme) during the period from January 1st through December 31st 2011 (RSCM 2012).

## iv) Estimation of sample size

During the period from January 1st to December 31st 2011, 20 billing administrators in the financial department were involved in the billing process for patients whose costs were reimbursed under the FFS method, and 13 billing administrators in the Patient Insurance Service Unit were involved in the billing process for patients whose costs were reimbursed under the casemix method. The sample size for this sub-study was 33 billing administrators (RSCM 2012).

## v) Sources of data

The data source for this study was the results of a perception questionnaire survey conducted with billing administrators in the financial department and the Patient Insurance Service Unit who were involved in the billing process.

## vi) Study tools

The study tools included a modified questionnaire with 5-point Likert-type scales based on Young's theory (Jamieson 2004, Landrum and Prybutok 2009). The questionnaire included 19 questions divided into 5 dimensions: tangibility (2 questions), reliability (6 questions), responsiveness (5 questions), assurance (3 questions), and empathy (3 questions) (Aryani and Rahmawati 2010, Landrum and Prybutok 2009). The questionnaire was tested in a similar national referral hospital in Jakarta with 20 respondents, and the results of the validity and reliability tests were as follows: $r_{table}=0.443$ with a 95% level of confidence (Gerstman 2015, Dahlan 2009). The $r_{test}$ for the questionnaire was 0.758, which was higher than the $r_{table}$ value ($r_{test}>r_{table}$). These results indicated that the questionnaire fulfilled the reliability test. The validity test for the questionnaire was calculated using SPSS version 22 with a 95% level of confidence.

Table 3.7 Validity test for the questionnaire on the perceptions of billing
administrators

| Questions | Validity Test | Memo |
|:---:|:---:|:---:|
| 1 | .456* | Valid |
| 2 | .610** | Valid |
| 3 | .695** | Valid |
| 4 | .695** | Valid |
| 5 | .747** | Valid |
| 6 | .826** | Valid |
| 7 | .888** | Valid |
| 8 | .888** | Valid |
| 9 | .610** | Valid |
| 10 | .425 | Valid |
| 11 | .716** | Valid |
| 12 | .601** | Valid |
| 13 | .687** | Valid |
| 14 | .727** | Valid |
| 15 | .697** | Valid |
| 16 | .734** | Valid |
| 17 | .697** | Valid |
| 18 | .695** | Valid |
| 19 | .734** | Valid |

Table 3.8 shows the results of the validity test for the
questionnaire, which were higher than the $r_{table}$ value, indicating
that the questionnaire fulfilled the validity test. Based on the
results of the reliability and validity tests, the questionnaire was
used to survey the perceptions of billing administrators.

## vii) Data collection

The survey was conducted in the financial department for billing administrators who used the FFS method and in the Patient Insurance Service Unit for billing administrators who used the casemix method. The respondents were informed about the survey and filled out a consent form. The respondents answered the questions in the questionnaire with a check mark (√). The score for each answer was based on the following grading system:

a.  The first answer   = 5
b.  The second answer = 4
c.  The third answer   = 3
d.  The fourth answer  = 2
e.  The fifth answer   = 1

These scores showed the respondents' perceptions of the billing process. Higher scores indicated less complexity in the billing process, and lower scores indicated more complexity in the billing process.

## viii) Data analysis

The 2 survey groups, FFS billing administrators and casemix billing administrators, were analysed following the same steps. The respondents' scores on the questions were aggregated into dimension scores. The score for each dimension was analysed by the descriptive method and the Kolmogorov-Smirnov test for normality. The comparison of each dimension's score between the two groups of billing administrators was conducted using t-tests with SPSS version 22 and 95% confidence levels (Pett 2016, Gerstman 2015, Dahlan 2009).

To describe the billing process under the FFS and casemix methods, the mean or median scores for each question were calculated and then linked back to the answers on the questionnaire.

The question responses described the billing administrators' perceptions of the billing process under the FFS and casemix methods. Then, those answers were arranged into the activities of the billing process to qualitatively show the differences in the billing process between the FFS and casemix methods.

## 3.5   Research Ethics

This study was approved by the Research Ethics Committee of Universiti Kebangsaan Malaysia, Cheras-Malaysia, Number UKM.FPR.4/244/UNU-2015-001 (appendices D and E); the Health Research Ethics Committee—Faculty of Medicine, Universitas Indonesia and Cipto Mangunkusumo Hospital, Jakarta, Indonesia, Number 709/UN2.FI/ETIK/IX/2014 ; and the Research Department of Cipto Mangunkusumo Hospital, Jakarta, Indonesia, Number LB.02.01/X.2/629/2014.

# IV RESULTS

## 4.1 Review of The Hospital's Annual Reports

In 2011, the site of study did not have the integrated information system. So, the researcher collected manually 26,526 of patients reimbursed by the FFS method from the patient registrations, the medical records, and the hospital claims. For 13,971 of patients reimbursed using the casemix method, the researcher collected data from INA-CBG's software, but many of data coloums were still blank and should be completed manually from the patient registrations. Collecting data manually was needed more time, moreover those data scattered among the medical services unit, the Patient Insurance Service Unit, the Medical Records unit, and the Finance Department.

For outpatient services, 22,643 patients' costs were reimbursed using the fee-for-service (FFS) method, and 9,584 patients' costs were reimbursed using the casemix method. For inpatient services, 3,883 patients' costs were reimbursed via FFS, and 4,387 patients' costs were reimbursed via casemix. In table 4.1, the largest age groups among patients whose costs were reimbursed using FFS were children aged 0-4 years (2,168 patients; 9.5%) and adults aged 45-49 years (2,157 patients; 9.5%) for outpatient services and children aged 0-4 years (612 patients; 15.8%) for inpatient services. The largest age groups among patients whose costs were reimbursed using the casemix method were children aged of 0-4 years (1,018 patients; 23.2%) for inpatient services and adults aged 45-49 years (925 patients; 9.7%) for outpatient services.

Table 4.1 Age distribution of patients whose costs were reimbursed under the FFS and casemix payment methods for outpatient and inpatient services in 2011

| Age Group* | FFS | | | | Casemix | | | |
|---|---|---|---|---|---|---|---|---|
| | Outpatient | | Inpatient | | Outpatient | | Inpatient | |
| | Fre quency | Percent (%) | Fre quency | Percent (%) | Fre quency | Percent (%) | Fre quency | Percent (%) |
| 0–4 | 2,168 | 9.5 | 612 | 15.8 | 462 | 4.8 | 1,018 | 23.2 |
| 5–9 | 1,452 | 6.4 | 338 | 8.7 | 805 | 8.4 | 197 | 4.5 |
| 10–14 | 1,304 | 5.8 | 145 | 3.7 | 861 | 9.0 | 143 | 3.3 |
| 15–19 | 1,166 | 5.2 | 166 | 4.3 | 905 | 9.4 | 275 | 6.3 |
| 20–24 | 1,306 | 5.8 | 225 | 5.8 | 500 | 5.2 | 418 | 9.5 |
| 25–29 | 1,612 | 7.1 | 255 | 6.6 | 630 | 6.6 | 530 | 12.1 |
| 30–34 | 1,344 | 6.0 | 249 | 6.4 | 590 | 6.2 | 505 | 11.5 |
| 35–39 | 1,586 | 7.0 | 318 | 8.2 | 805 | 8.4 | 417 | 9.5 |
| 40–44 | 1,816 | 8.0 | 330 | 8.5 | 749 | 7.8 | 266 | 6.0 |
| 45–49 | 2,157 | 9.5 | 317 | 8.2 | 925 | 9.7 | 206 | 4.7 |
| 50–54 | 2,125 | 9.4 | 301 | 7.8 | 869 | 9.1 | 222 | 5.0 |
| 55–59 | 1,716 | 7.5 | 253 | 6.5 | 584 | 6.1 | 134 | 3.1 |
| 60–64 | 1,362 | 6.0 | 149 | 3.8 | 424 | 4.4 | 29 | 0.7 |
| 65–69 | 843 | 3.7 | 109 | 2.7 | 290 | 3.0 | 18 | 0.4 |
| 70–74 | 449 | 2.0 | 68 | 1.8 | 185 | 1.9 | 9 | 0.2 |
| 75+ | 237 | 1.1 | 48 | 1.2 | | | | |
| Total | 22,643 | 100.0 | 3,883 | 100.0 | 9,584 | 100.0 | 4,387 | 100.0 |

*Based on The Indonesian Health Profile 2016 (MOH 2017)

Table 4.2 Gender distribution of patients whose costs were reimbursed under the FFS and casemix payment methods for outpatient and inpatient services in 2011

| Gender | FFS | | | | Casemix | | | |
|---|---|---|---|---|---|---|---|---|
| | Outpatient | | Inpatient | | Outpatient | | Inpatient | |
| | Freuency | Percent (%) | Frequency | Percent (%) | Frequency | Percent (%) | Frequency | Percent (%) |
| Male | 11,205 | 49.5 | 1,670 | 43.0 | 4,006 | 41.8 | 1,291 | 29.4 |
| Female | 11,438 | 50.5 | 2,213 | 57.0 | 5,578 | 58.2 | 3,096 | 70.6 |
| Total | 22,643 | 100.0 | 3,883 | 100.0 | 9,584 | 100.0 | 4,387 | 100.0 |

Table 4.2 shows that a larger proportion of the patients whose costs were reimbursed using the FFS method and the casemix method were female. A total of 11,438 female patients (50.5%) used FFS for outpatient services, and 2,213 female patients (57.0%) used FFS for inpatient services. In addition, 5,578 female patients (58.2%) used casemix for outpatient services, and 3,096 female patients (70.6%) used casemix for inpatient services.

In table 4.3, the West Java area had the most referrals among patients whose costs were reimbursed under the casemix method: 1,582 inpatient cases (36.1%) and 5,858 outpatient cases (61.1%). A total of 1,119 inpatient cases (25.5%) and 338 outpatient cases (3.5%) were referred from Jakarta province. Since the Jaminan Persalinan (Jampersal, maternity insurance) programme was launched in May 2011 by the Ministry of Health (MOH) as an improvement to the Jamkesmas programme, Jakarta citizens have been allowed to participate in the maternity insurance programme. The provinces of West Java, Banten and Lampung directly border Jakarta province—the location of the study site. Those three provinces represent the three highest referring areas for patients whose costs were reimbursed using the casemix method.

Table 4.3 Referral area distribution of patients whose costs were reimbursed under the casemix payment method for inpatient and outpatient services in 2011

| Inpatient | | | Outpatient | | |
|---|---|---|---|---|---|
| Referral Area | Fre quency | Percent | Referral Area | Fre quency | Percent |
| West Java | 1,582 | 36.1 | West Java | 5,858 | 61.1 |
| DKI Jakarta | 1,119 | 25.5 | Banten | 1,749 | 18.2 |
| Banten | 688 | 15.7 | Lampung | 872 | 9.1 |
| Lampung | 442 | 10.1 | DKI Jakarta | 338 | 3.5 |
| Central Java | 156 | 3.6 | Central Java | 273 | 2.8 |
| Bengkulu | 78 | 1.8 | Bengkulu | 107 | 1.1 |
| West Kalimantan | 40 | 0.9 | Papua | 56 | 0.6 |
| Papua | 33 | 0.8 | Maluku | 53 | 0.6 |
| Riau | 32 | 0.7 | Riau | 45 | 0.5 |
| Maluku | 31 | 0.7 | Jambi | 38 | 0.4 |
| Others (North Sulawesi, East Nusa Tenggara, etc.) | 186 | 4.3 | Others (North Sumatera, East Java, etc.) | 195 | 2.0 |
| Total | 4,387 | 100.0 | | 9,584 | 100.0 |

Table 4.4 Referral area distribution of patients whose costs under the FFS payment method for inpatient and outpatient services in 2011

| Referral Area | Inpatient | | Outpatient | |
|---|---|---|---|---|
| | Frequency | Percent | Frequency | Percent |
| East Jakarta | 1,267 | 32.6 | 6,846 | 30.2 |
| Central Jakarta | 1,014 | 26.1 | 6,082 | 26.9 |
| South Jakarta | 630 | 16.2 | 3,391 | 15.0 |
| West Jakarta | 571 | 14.7 | 3,321 | 14.7 |
| North Jakarta | 386 | 10.0 | 2,975 | 13.1 |
| Homeless | 12 | 0.3 | 0 | - |
| Seribu Islands | 3 | 0.1 | 28 | 0.1 |
| Total | 3,883 | 100.0 | 22,643 | 100.00 |

As seen in table 4.4, East Jakarta had the highest number of referrals for patients reimbursed using the FFS method with 1,267 inpatient cases (32.6%) and 6,846 outpatient cases (30.2%). Central Jakarta—where the study site was located—had 1,014 inpatient cases (26.1%) and 6,082 outpatient cases (26.9%). There were no referral areas outside Jakarta province because the Gakin programme was only for Jakarta citizens.

Table 4.5 Primary diagnosis distribution of patients whose costs were reimbursed under the FFS payment method according to ICD-10 codes for outpatient services in 2011

| ICD-10 Codes | Description | Frequency | Percent |
|---|---|---|---|
| Z00–Z99.9 | Factors influencing health status and contact with health services | 11,403 | 50.4 |
| V01–Y98.9 | External causes of morbidity and mortality | 6,250 | 27.6 |
| C00–D48.9 | Neoplasms | 757 | 3.3 |
| I00–I99.9 | Diseases of the circulatory system | 608 | 2.7 |
| D50–D89.9 | Diseases of blood and blood-forming organs and certain disorders involving the immune mechanisms | 528 | 2.3 |
| A00–B99.9 | Certain infectious and parasitic diseases | 502 | 2.2 |
| E00–E90.9 | Endocrine, nutritional and metabolic diseases | 494 | 2.2 |
| H00–H59.9 | Diseases of the eye and adnexa | 332 | 1.5 |
| N00–N99.9 | Diseases of the genitourinary system | 325 | 1.4 |
| ...continuation | | | |
| M00-M99.9 | Diseases of the musculoskeletal system and connective tissue | 292 | 1.3 |
| Others (F00-F99.9; G00–G99.9; etc.) | — | 1,152 | 5.1 |
| | Total | 22,643 | 100.0 |

Table 4.6 Primary diagnosis distribution of patients whose costs were reimbursed under the casemix payment method according to ICD-10 codes for outpatient services in 2011

| ICD-10 Codes | Description | Frequency | Percent |
|---|---|---|---|
| Z00–Z99.9 | Factors influencing health status and contact with health services | 8,143 | 85.0 |
| C00–D48.9 | Neoplasms | 405 | 4.2 |
| E00–E89.9 | Endocrine, nutritional and metabolic diseases | 257 | 2.7 |
| I00–I99.9 | Diseases of the circulatory system | 203 | 2.1 |
| N00–N99.9 | Diseases of the genitourinary system | 164 | 1.7 |
| Q00–Q99.9 | Congenital malformations, deformations and chromosomal abnormalities | 103 | 1.1 |
| A00–B99.9 | Certain infectious and parasitic diseases | 73 | 0.8 |
| M00–M99 | Diseases of the musculoskeletal system and connective tissue | 60 | 0.6 |
| R00–R99.9 | Symptoms, signs, and abnormal clinical and laboratory findings not classified elsewhere | 58 | 0.6 |
| Others (G00–99.9; K00–K99.9; S00–S99.9) | Others | 118 | 1.2 |
| | Total | 9,584 | 100.0 |

Table 4.5 and table 4.6 show that the most common primary diagnosis for outpatient services was factors influencing health status and contact with health services (Z00–Z99.9): 11,403 patients (50.4%) under the FFS payment method and 8,143 patients (85.0%) under the casemix payment method. Additionally, several other diagnoses were prevalent in both groups, such as neoplasms, endocrine, nutritional and metabolic diseases, diseases of the circulatory system, and certain infectious and parasitic diseases.

Table 4.7 Primary diagnosis distribution of patients whose costs were reimbursed under the FFS payment method according to ICD-10 codes for inpatient services in 2011

| ICD-10 Codes | Descriptions | Number of Patients | Percent |
|---|---|---|---|
| C00–D48.9 | Neoplasms | 722 | 18.6 |
| O00–O99.9 | Pregnancy, childbirth, puerperium | 599 | 15.4 |
| P00–P96.9 | Certain conditions originating in the perinatal period | 521 | 13.4 |
| I00–I99.9 | Diseases of the circulatory system | 343 | 8.8 |
| A00–B99.9 | Certain infectious and parasitic diseases | 288 | 7.5 |
| Z00–Z99.9 | Factors influencing health status and contact with health services | 277 | 7.1 |
| K00–K99.9 | Diseases of the digestive system | 240 | 6.2 |
| S00–T98.9 | Injury, poisoning and certain other consequences of external causes | 226 | 5.8 |
| H00–H59.9 | Diseases of the eye and adnexa | 199 | 5.1 |
| D50–D89 | Diseases of blood and blood-forming organs and certain disorders involving the immune mechanisms | 190 | 4.9 |
| Others (J00–J99.9; N00–N99.9; L00–L99.9) | | 278 | 7.2 |
| | Total | 3,883 | 100.0 |

Table 4.8 Primary diagnosis distribution of patients whose costs were reimbursed under the casemix payment method according to ICD-10 codes for inpatient services in 2011

| ICD-10 Codes | Descriptions | Number of Patients | Percent |
|---|---|---|---|
| O00–O99.9 | Pregnancy, childbirth, puerperium | 1,584 | 36.1 |
| P00–P96.9 | Certain conditions originating in the perinatal period | 764 | 17.4 |
| Z00–Z99.9 | Factors influencing health status and contact with health services | 558 | 12.7 |
| C00–D48.9 | Neoplasms | 366 | 8.3 |
| Q00–Q99.9 | Congenital malformations, deformations and chromosomal abnormalities | 221 | 5.0 |
| D50–D89.9 | Diseases of blood and blood-forming organs and certain disorders involving the immune mechanisms | 191 | 4.4 |
| I00–I99.9 | Diseases of the circulatory system | 136 | 3.1 |
| K00–K93.9 | Diseases of the digestive system | 99 | 2.3 |
| H00–H59.9 | Diseases of the eye and adnexa | 89 | 2.0 |
| N00–N 99.9 | Diseases of the genitourinary system | 64 | 1.5 |
| S00–S99.9; J00–J99.9; etc. | Others | 315 | 7.2 |
| | Total | 4,387 | 100.0 |

Table 4.7 shows that the most common primary diagnoses for inpatient services among patients using the FFS method were neoplasms (722 patients; 18.6%) and pregnancy, childbirth, puerperium (599 patients; 15.4%). As seen in table 4.8, the most common primary diagnoses among patients using the casemix method were pregnancy, childbirth, puerperium (1,584 patients; 36.1%) and certain conditions originating in the perinatal period (764 patients; 17.4%), which were covered under the maternity insurance programme. Patients whose costs were reimbursed using the FFS method and those whose costs were reimbursed using the casemix method had several of the same primary diagnoses, such as certain conditions originating in the perinatal period, diseases of the circulatory system, and diseases of the eye and adnexa.

## 4.2 Review of Medical Services

### 4.2.1 Review of Medical Records

#### a. Medical record review of outpatient services

In the Indonesian health security system, policlinics provide medical care such as consultations, laboratory services, radiology examinations, and pharmacy services, and patients are able to visit several services in the same day. Table 4.9 shows that Nineteen main policlinics and 4 main supporting units provided services for the two groups of patients in this study.

Table 4.9 Policlinics and medical supporting units for patients whose costs were reimbursed under the FFS and casemix payment methods in 2011

| No. | Policlinics / Services Units |
|:---:|---|
| 1 | Laboratory |
| 2 | Pharmacy |
| 3 | Radiology |
| 4 | Blood Transfusion Unit |
| 5 | General Surgery |
| 6 | Paediatric |
| 7 | Internal Diseases |
| 8 | Haemodialysis |
| 9 | Radiotherapy |
| 10 | Medical Rehabilitation |
| 11 | Ophthalmology |
| 12 | ENT |
| 13 | Neurology |
| 14 | Obstetrics and Gynaecology |
| 15 | Thalassemia |
| 16 | Cardiology |
| 17 | Psychiatry |
| 18 | Dermatology and Venereology |
| 19 | Urology |
| 20 | Neurosurgery |
| 21 | Dental Clinics |
| 22 | Nutrition |
| 23 | Acupuncture |

Sources: The Cipto Mangunkusumo Hospital Report 2011. (The Planning and Develpoment Department of RSCM 2012)

Among the outpatients, 22,643 patients' costs were reimbursed using the FFS method, and 9,584 patients' costs were reimbursed using the casemix method. The five most common diagnoses were selected as the samples for this sub-study (table 4.10). A total of 5,914 patients under the FFS method (26.1%) and 3,923 patients under the casemix method (40.9%) were selected based on the five most common diagnoses for outpatient services.

Table 4.10 The five most common diagnoses for outpatient services among patients whose costs were reimbursed under the FFS and casemix payment methods

| No | ICD-10 | | INA-CBG Codes | | FFS | Casemix |
|---|---|---|---|---|---|---|
| | Codes | Descriptions | Codes | Descriptions | | |
| 1 | Z09.8 | Follow-up examination after other treatment for other conditions | Q-5-44 | Other non-complex chronic condition | 3,785 | 1,840 |
| 2 | Z08.9 | Follow-up examination after unspecified treatment for malignant neoplasm | Q-5-44 | Other non-complex chronic condition | 1,321 | 1,787 |
| 3 | B24 | Unspecified human immunodeficiency virus (HIV) disease | Q-5-34 | Human immunodeficiency virus infection | 348 | 38 |
| 4 | Z48.8 | Other specified surgical follow-up care | Q-5-44 | Other non-complex chronic condition | 344 | 119 |
| 5 | Z49.1 | Extracorporeal dialysis | N-3-15 | Dialysis | 116 | 139 |
| | | Total | | | 5,914 | 3,923 |

To fulfil the study objectives, this sub-study compared the hospital charges for the five most common diagnoses between patients using FFS and those using casemix.

### i) Follow-up examination after other treatment for other conditions with other non-complex chronic condition (ICD-10 code Z09.8; INA-CBG code Q-5-44)

A total of 3,785 patients under FFS and 1,840 patients under casemix had ICD-10 code Z09.8. The median charge under the FFS method was IDR 420,000 (min–max IDR 22,430–8,843,000), which was higher than that under the casemix method (IDR 325,575), and the difference was significant at p=0.0001.

Table 4. 11 Comparison of hospital charges in the outpatient services for follow-up examination after other treatment for other conditions with other non-complex chronic condition (Z09.8; Q-5-44) between patients whose costs were reimbursed under the FFS and casemix payment methods

| Variable | Type of Payment | | p |
|---|---|---|---|
| | FFS (IDR) Median (Min–max) | Casemix (IDR) Median | |
| Hospital Charge | 420,000 (22,430–8,843,000) | 325,575 | 0.0001* |

* Two-Independent- Samples Test.

### ii) Follow-up examination after unspecified treatment for malignant neoplasm with other non-complex chronic condition (ICD-10 code Z08.9; INA-CBG code Q-5-44)

There were 1,321 patients under FFS and 1,787 patients under casemix with ICD-10 code Z08.9. The median for the FFS method was IDR 650,000 (min–max IDR 300,000–9,850,576), which was higher than the median for the casemix method (IDR 325,575), and the difference was significant at p=0.0001.

Table 4.12 Comparison of hospital charges in the outpatient services for follow-up examination after unspecified treatment for malignant with other non-complex chronic condition(Z08.9; Q-5-44) between patients whose costs were reimbursed under the FFS and casemix payment methods

| Variable | Type of Payment | | p |
|---|---|---|---|
| | FFS (IDR) Median (Min–max) | Casemix (IDR) Median | |
| Hospital Charge | 650,000 (300,000–9,850,576) | 325,575 | 0.0001* |

* Two-Independent- Samples Test.

### iii) Unspecified human immunodeficiency virus (HIV) disease (ICD-10 code B24; INA-CBG code Q-5-34)

A total of 348 patients under FFS and 38 patients under casemix had ICD-10 code B-24. The median charge under the FFS method was IDR 460,000 (min–max IDR 409,750–1,847,720), which was higher than the median charge under the casemix method (IDR 452,551). The difference in the median hospital charge between patients under FFS and those under casemix was significant at p=0.0001.

Table 4.13 Comparison of hospital charges in the outpatient services for unspecified human immunodeficiency virus (B24; Q-5-34) between patients whose costs were reimbursed under the FFS and casemix payment methods

| Variable | Type of Payment | | p |
|---|---|---|---|
| | FFS (IDR) Median (Min–max) | Casemix (IDR) Median | |
| Hospital Charge | 460,000 (409,750–1,847,720) | 452,551 | 0.0001* |

* Two-Independent- Samples Test.

### iv) Other specified surgical follow-up care with other non-complex chronic condition (ICD-10 code Z48.8; INA-CBG code Q-5-44)

There were 344 patients under FFS and 119 patients under casemix with ICD-10 code Z48.8. The median charge under the FFS method was IDR 425,500 (min–max IDR 273,710–1,027,000), which was higher than the median charge under the casemix method (IDR 325,575). The difference in the median hospital charge between patients under FFS and those under casemix was significant at p=0.0001.

Table 4.14 Comparison of hospital charges in the outpatient services for other specified surgical follow-up care with other non-complex chronic condition (Z48.8; Q-5-44) between patients whose costs were reimbursed under the FFS and casemix payment methods

| Variable | Type of Payment | | p |
|---|---|---|---|
| | FFS (IDR) Median (Min–max) | Casemix (IDR) Median | |
| Hospital Charge | 425,500 (273,710–1,027,000) | 325,575 | 0.0001* |

* Two-Independent- Samples Test.

### v) Extracorporeal dialysis (ICD-10 code Z49.1; INA-CBG code N-3-15)

A total of 116 patients under FFS and 139 patients under casemix had ICD-10 code Z49.1. The median charge under the FFS method was IDR 1,271,558 (min–max 951,350–1,936,720), which is higher than the median charge under the casemix method (IDR 1,178,556). The hospital charge for extracorporeal dialysis was significantly different between patients whose costs were reimbursed using FFS and casemix at p=0.0001.

Table 4.15 Comparison of hospital charges in the outpatient services for extracorporeal dialysis(Z49.1; N-3-15) between patients whose costs were reimbursed under the FFS and casemix payment methods

| Variable | Type of Payment | | p |
|---|---|---|---|
| | FFS (IDR)) Median (Min–max | Casemix (IDR) Median | |
| Hospital Charge | 1,271,558 (951,350–1,936,720) | 1,178,556 | 0.0001* |

* Two-Independent- Samples Test.

The median charge for extracorporeal dialysis under FFS was IDR 1,271,558 (min–max 951,350–1,936,720), which was higher than the median charge for patients under the casemix payment method (IDR 1,178,556). The hospital charge for extracorporeal dialysis was significantly different between patients whose costs were reimbursed using FFS and casemix at p=0.0001.

The statistical calculations for the five most common diagnoses listed above showed that all the comparisons of hospital charges between patients reimbursed using the FFS and casemix methods were significantly different at p=0.0001. The median hospital charges for patients with one of the five most common diagnoses were lower under the casemix method than under the FFS method.

## b. Medical record review of inpatient services

For the medical review of inpatient services, the five most common services were selected for patients under FFS and casemix. The hospital charges for the five most common diagnoses were compared between patients whose costs were reimbursed using FFS and patients whose costs were reimbursed using casemix. A total of 3,883 patients in public wards were discharged by doctors under the FFS method, and 4,387 patients in public wards were discharged under the casemix method. The five most common diagnoses were selected for the sample: 984 patients (25.3%) under the FFS method and 1,373 patients under the casemix method (31.3%).

Table 4.16 Five most common diagnoses for inpatient services among patients whose costs were reimbursed under the FFS and casemix payment methods

| No | ICD-10 | | CBG Codes | | | |
| | Codes | Descriptions | Codes | Descriptions | FFS | Casemix |
|---|---|---|---|---|---|---|
| 1 | O82.9 | Caesarean delivery | O-6-10 | Inpatient procedures (IP) caesarean delivery | 248 | 497 |
| 2 | P03.4 | Foetus and newborn affected by caesarean delivery | P-8-17 | Inpatient medical (IM) neonate, birth weight > 2,499 grams | 219 | 136 |
| 3 | Z51.1 | Chemotherapy session for neoplasm | C-4-13 | Inpatient medical (IM) chemotherapy | 210 | 358 |
| 4 | O80.9 | Single spontaneous delivery | O-6-13 | Inpatient medical (IM) vaginal delivery | 192 | 280 |
| 5 | C53.9 | Malignant neoplasm of cervix uteri | W-4-10 | Inpatient female reproductive system malignancy | 115 | 102 |
| | | Total | | | 984 | 1,373 |

This objective of this sub-study was to determine whether hospital charge and length of stay (LOS) were higher for patients whose costs were reimbursed via FFS than for patients whose costs were reimbursed via casemix. To fulfil the objective of this study, LOS and hospital charge for the five most common diagnoses were compared for patients using the FFS and casemix methods.

## i) Caesarean delivery (ICD-10 code O82.9; INA-CBG code O-6-10)

There were 248 patients with caesarean delivery under FFS, and 497 patients under casemix. The comparison of LOS and hospital charge between the two groups of patients is below:

Table 4.17 Comparison of LOS and hospital charges in the inpatient services for caesareandelivery (O82.9; O-6-10) between patients whose costs were reimbursed under the FFS and casemix payment methods

| Variable | Median (Min–max) | | p |
| --- | --- | --- | --- |
| | FFS | Casemix | |
| LOS (Days) | 6.0 (4–13) | 5.5 (5.5–7.5) | 0.0001* |
| Hospital Charge (IDR) | 5,404,807 (1,535,000– 46,531,168) | 5,291,100 (4,766,102–6,520,427) | 0.0001* |

* Mann-Whitney U test; LOS=length of stay.

Significant differences were found between the FFS and casemix payment methods with respect to median LOS and hospital charge for caesarean delivery (O82.9; O-6-10) at p=0.0001. The median LOS and hospital charge for caesarean delivery under FFS (6.0 days; IDR 5,404,807) were higher than the median LOS and hospital charge under casemix (5.5 days; IDR 5,291,100).

## ii) Foetus and newborn affected by caesarean delivery with neonate, birth weight > 2,499 grams (ICD-10 code P03.4; INA-CBG code P-8-17)

There were 219 patients under FFS and 136 patients under casemix categorized as foetus and newborn affected by caesarean delivery with neonate, birth weight > 2,499 grams (P03.4; P-8-17). The comparison between the two groups of patients was conducted using statistical analysis.

Table 4.18 Comparison of LOS and hospital charges in the inpatient
services for foetus and newborn affected by caesarean delivery
with neonate, birth weight > 2,499 grams (P03.4; P-8-17)
between patients whose costs were reimbursed under the FFS
and casemix payment methods

| Variable | Median (Min–max) | | p |
| --- | --- | --- | --- |
| | FFS | Casemix | |
| LOS (Days) | 5.0 (3.0–25.0) | 4.2 (4.2–13.1) | 0.0001* |
| Hospital Charge (IDR) | 11,450,444 (2,036,585– 74,070,754) | 2,951,414 (2,951,414– 19,823,927) | 0.0001* |

* Mann-Whitney U test; LOS=length of stay.

The differences in the median LOS and hospital charge
between the FFS and casemix payment methods were significant at
p=0.0001. The median LOS and hospital charge for this common
diagnosis for patients whose costs were reimbursed using FFS (5.0
days; IDR 11,450,444) were higher than the median LOS and
hospital charge for patients whose costs were reimbursed using
casemix (4.2 days; IDR 2,951,414).

iii) **Chemotherapy session for neoplasm (ICD-10 code Z51.1;
INA-CBG code C-4-13)**

A total of 210 patients under FFS and 358 patients under
casemix were categorized as having a chemotherapy session for
neoplasm. Significant differences between the FFS and casemix
payment methods were found for median LOS and hospital
charge for chemotherapy session for neoplasm (Z51.1; C-4-
13) at p=0.0001. The median LOS and hospital charge for a
chemotherapy session for neoplasm were higher for patients whose
costs were reimbursed using FFS (5.0 days; IDR 6,546,876) than
for patients whose costs were reimbursed using casemix (4.6 days;
IDR 3,205,631).

Table 4.19 Comparison of LOS and hospital charges in the inpatient
services for chemotherapy session for neoplasm (Z51.1; C-4-
13) between patients whose costs were reimbursed under the
FFS and casemix payment methods

| Variable | Median (Min–max) | | p |
|---|---|---|---|
| | FFS | Casemix | |
| LOS (Days) | 5.0 (3.0–45.0) | 4.6 (4.6–12.0) | 0.0001* |
| Hospital Charge (IDR) | 6,546,876 (2,071,004–93,451,728) | 3,205,631 (3,205,631–8,311,329) | 0.0001* |

* Mann-Whitney U test; LOS=length of stay.

## iv) Single spontaneous delivery (ICD-10 code O80.9; INA-CBG code O-6-13)

A total of 192 patients under FFS and 280 patients under
casemix were categorized as having a single spontaneous delivery.
Median LOS and hospital charge for single spontaneous delivery
were significantly different between patients using FFS and
patients using casemix at p=0.0001. Median LOS and hospital
charge for patients having a single spontaneous delivery (O80.9)
were higher under the FFS method (5.0 days; IDR 4,890,022)
than under the casemix payment method (3.9 days; 2,613,718).

Table 4.20 Comparison of LOS and hospital charges in the inpatient
services for single spontaneous delivery (O80.9; O-6-13)
between patients whose costs were reimbursed under the FFS
and casemix payment methods

| Variable | Median (Min–max) | | p |
|---|---|---|---|
| | FFS | Casemix | |
| LOS (Days) | 5.0 (3.0–12.0) | 3.9 (3.9–8.0) | 0.0001* |
| Hospital Charge (IDR) | 4,890,022 (2,086,153–14,669,732) | 2,613,718 (2,613,718–5,709,812) | 0.0001* |

* Mann-Whitney U test; LOS=length of stay.

## v) Malignant neoplasm of cervix uteri (ICD-10 Code C53.9; INA-CBG code W-4-10)

There were 115 patients under FFS and 102 patients under casemix with malignant neoplasm of cervix uteri (C53.9; W-4-10). The hospital charge for the two groups of patients were compared by statistical analysis. Median LOS and hospital charge for patients with malignant neoplasm of cervix uteri were significantly different for patients using FFS and patients using casemix at p=0.0001. Median LOS and hospital charge for malignant neoplasm of cervix uteri were higher under FFS (10.0 days; IDR 13,170,730) than under casemix (8.3 days; IDR 8,756,115).

Table 4.21 Comparison of LOS and hospital charges in the inpatient services for malignant neoplasm of cervix uteri between patients whose costs were reimbursed under the FFS and casemix payment methods

| Variable | Median (Min–max) | | p |
| --- | --- | --- | --- |
| | FFS | Casemix | |
| LOS (Days) | 10.0 (4.0–32.0) | 8.3 (6.1–13.8) | 0.0001* |
| Hospital Charge (IDR) | 13,170,730 (2,273,353–148,230,898) | 8,756,115 (6,478,275–15,740,105) | 0.0001* |

* Mann-Whitney U test; LOS=length of stay.

Based on the 5 statistical analyses described above, this study observed significant differences between patients under FFS and patients under casemix in terms of hospital charges for all five of the most common diagnoses for outpatients at p=0.0001. In addition, LOS and hospital charge for all five of the most common diagnoses for inpatients were significantly different between patients whose costs were casemix method (p=0.0001). Median hospital charge and LOS for the five most common diagnoses were lower under the casemix method than under the FFS method.

## 4.2.2 Review of Unnecessary Admissions

A total of 357 patients had a one-day hospitalization in 2011 under the FFS scheme, and of those patients, 257 (72.0%) had an unnecessary admission, while 100 had a necessary admission. A total of 407 patients had a one-day hospitalization in 2011 under the casemix scheme, and of those patients, 157 (38.6%) had an unnecessary admission, while 250 had a necessary admission. The patients with unnecessary admissions whose costs were reimbursed through the FFS method were Jakarta citizens, and those whose costs were paid through the casemix method were citizens of other provinces.

Table 4.22 Comparison of the proportion of unnecessarily admitted patients whose costs were reimbursed under the FFS and casemix methods in 2011

| Type of Payment | Unnecessary Admission (N,%) | Necessary Admission (N,%) | p |
|---|---|---|---|
| FFS | 257 (72.0%) | 100 (28.0%) | 0.0001* |
| Casemix | 157 (38.6%) | 250 (61.4%) | |
| Total | 404 | 350 | |

* Chi-square test.

Of the 357 patients under the FFS method and the 407 patients under the casemix method who were admitted to the emergency room or a third-class ward for a one-day hospitalization, 257 (72.0%) and 157 (38.6%), respectively, were admitted unnecessarily. There was a significant difference in the proportion of unnecessary admissions between patients under the FFS method and patients under the casemix method in 2011 (p=0.0001). Patients whose costs were reimbursed via the FFS method were 4.092 times more likely to have an unnecessary admission than patients whose costs were reimbursed via casemix. The unnecessary admission rate among patients under the FFS method was 1.87 times higher than the rate among patients under the casemix method (72.0%;38.6%, p=0.0001).

Patients who were unnecessarily admitted under both payment methods were mostly female (FFS=166; 64.6% and casemix=124; 79.0%). The largest proportion of patients in both payment groups were in the 40-50 year age range. Patients from both the FFS and casemix groups who had an unnecessary admission came from low-income families with a public ward (3rd-class ward) health insurance benefit package.

Table 4.23 Distribution of gender and age among patients with unnecessary admissions whose costs were reimbursed under the FFS and casemix payment methods in 2011

| Items | Fee-for-service (N=257) (n,%) | Casemix (N=157) (n,%) |
|---|---|---|
| **Gender:** | | |
| Male | 91(35.4%) | 33 (21.0%) |
| Female | 166 (64.6%) | 124 (79.0%) |
| **Age (years):** | | |
| 0–10 | 28 (10.9%) | 4 (2.6%) |
| 10–20 | 27 (10.5%) | 6 (3.8%) |
| 20–30 | 21 (8.2%) | 13 (8.3%) |
| 30–40 | 33 (12.8%) | 32 (20.4%) |
| 40–50 | 69 (26.9%) | 55 (35.0%) |
| 50–60 | 53 (20.6%) | 44 (28.0%) |
| 60–70 | 26 (10.1%) | 3 (1.9%) |

Table 4.24 Comparison of hospital charges for unnecessary admission between patients whose cost were reimbursed under the FFS and casemix payment methods in 2011

| Field | N | Median (IDR)** | Min-Max (IDR) | p |
|---|---|---|---|---|
| **FFS** | 257 | 3,895,850 | 407,500– 22,640,463 | 0,027* |
| **Casemix** | 157 | 3,600,514 | 2,866,618– 8,311,329 | |

* Mann-Whitney-U test

Differences were found between patients whose costs were reimbursed by FFS and those whose costs were reimbursed by casemix regarding hospital charges for unnecessary admissions (p=0.027). The median hospital charge was higher under the FFS method (IDR 3,895,850 min–max IDR 407,500–22,640,463) than under the casemix method (IDR 3,600,514 min–max IDR 2,866,618–8,311,329).

In the referral system, several grades were used when referring patients with a referral letter from a previous hospital to a referral hospital. To compare referral letter usage for casemix and FFS, the proportion of patients unnecessarily admitted to the hospital with a referral letter was analysed.

Table 4.25 Comparison of the proportion of referral letters in unnecessary admissions between the FFS and casemix payment methods

| Type of Payment | Without Referral Letter (N,%) | With Referral Letter (N,%) | p |
|---|---|---|---|
| FFS | 94 (36.6%) | 163 (63.4%) | 0.0001* |
| Casemix | 2 (1.4%) | 155 (98.7%) | |
| Total | 96 | 318 | |

* Chi-square test.

Referral letters from a previous lower-level health facility were used by only 163 patients (63.4%) in the FFS group who had an unnecessary admission, and the remaining 36.6% (94 patients) of unnecessary admissions were directly admitted to the emergency room without a referral letter. However, among patients in the casemix group, 155 patients (98.7%) had a referral letter from a lower-level health facility, and only 2 patients (1.3%) did not have a referral letter. There was a significant difference between patients whose costs were reimbursed via FFS and patients whose costs were reimbursed via casemix in terms of the proportion of patients who were admitted with and without referral letters (p=0.0001). The unnecessary admission rate without a referral letter was 28.2 times higher for patients under the FFS method than for patients under the casemix method (36.6%;1.3%, p=0.0001).

## 4.2.3 Logistic Regression Analysis of The Review of Medical Services

The review of medical services consisted of 2 sub-studies, i.e., a review of patients' medical records for the five most common diagnoses and a review of unnecessary admissions. Eight variables were included in both sub-studies, namely, type of payment, hospital charge, LOS, gender, age, type of case, type of service and unnecessary admission in the multiple logistic regression analysis model.

Correlations represent the most useful measure of association between two or more variables. Expressed in a single number called a correlation coefficient (r), correlations provide information about the direction (either positive or negative) and intensity (-1.0 to +1.0) of a relationship. Spearman's correlation tests were conducted on the variables, and the results are shown below:

Table 4.26 Correlation test on the review of medical services

| Variables | Correlation Coefficient (r) | p* |
|---|---|---|
| Type of Payment | | |
| Hospital Charge | -0.638 | 0.0001 |
| LOS | -0.490 | 0.0001 |
| Gender | -0.296 | 0.0001 |
| Age | -0.205 | 0.0001 |
| Type of Case | -0.438 | 0.0001 |
| Type of Service | -0.244 | 0.0001 |
| Unnecessary Admission | -0.369 | 0.0001 |

*Spearman's test.

Table 4.26 shows that all the variables were significantly correlated with type of payment at p=0.0001: gender, age and type of case exhibited weak correlations; LOS, type of case and unnecessary admission showed rather moderate correlations; and hospital charge exhibited a strong correlation. Based on this correlation analysis, all the independent variables were included in the logistic regression analysis model.

Regression analysis is performed to study the dependence of one variable—the dependent variable—on one or more other variables—the independent variables (Dahlan 2009). The dependent variable was type of payment, which is binary, i.e., FFS and casemix. And the independent variables were LOS, hospital charge, type of case, type of service, gender, age and unnecessary admission. For this study, the researcher selected binary logistic regression for the analysis with codes for the dependent and independent variables as follows:

Table 4.27 Codes for the dependent and independent variables in the multiple logistic regressionanalysis of the review of medical services

| No | Variable | Codes |
|----|----------|-------|
| 1 | Type of Payment | 0: FFS<br>1: Casemix |
| 2 | LOS | Continuous variable |
| 3 | Hospital Charge | Continuous variable |
| 4 | Type of Case | 0: Medical Case<br>1: Surgical Case |
| 5 | Type of Service | 0: Outpatient<br>1: Inpatient |
| 6 | Gender | 0: Male<br>1: Female |
| 7 | Age | Continuous variable |
| 8 | Unnecessary Admission | 0: Necessary Admission<br>1: Unnecessary Admission |

The omnibus test determined that the goodness of fit of the multiple logistic regression model was significant (p=0.0001). Thus, Ho was rejected, and Ha was accepted. This result indicates that all the independent variables (hospital charge, LOS, gender, age, type of case, type of service, and unnecessary admission), or a minimum of one independent variable, exhibited a significant association with the dependent variable (type of payment: the FFS method and the casemix method) at p=0.0001. In addition, the

Nagelkerke's $R^2$ value was 0.508, indicating that those independent variables influenced 50.8% of the variance of the dependent variable (type of payment).

Table 4.28 Odds ratios of independent variables associated with type of payment (FFS=0 and casemix=1)

| Variables | B | Wald | OR (95% CI) | p |
|---|---|---|---|---|
| Hospital Charge | -0.080 | 1,381.4 | 1.387 (1.079 – 1.389) | 0.0001* |
| LOS | -0.053 | 6.888 | 1.255 (1.014-1.297) | 0.009* |
| Gender (Male=0; Female=1) | -0.198 | 14.817 | 1.219 (1.103 – 1.348) | 0.0001* |
| Age | -0.013 | 104.816 | 1.127 (1.010 – 1.274) | 0.0001* |
| Type of Case (Medical=0; Surgical=1) | -1.531 | 254.870 | 4.630 (3.831 – 5.587) | 0.0001* |
| Type of Service (Outpatient=0; Inpatient=1) | -3.686 | 879.988 | 4.000 (3.125 – 5.000) | 0.0001* |
| Unnecessary Admission (Necessary admission=0; Unnecessary admission=1) | -0.844 | 53.591 | 2.326 (1.855 – 2.915) | 0.0001* |

Based on the results of the table above, the researcher has interpreted the odds ratio of the multiple logistic regression analysis on the review of medical service as follows:

1. Hospital charges for patients of the teaching hospital under the casemix method were found to be 1.387 times less than those of patients of the teaching hospital under the FFS method.
2. Patients of the teaching hospital whose costs were reimbursed under the casemix method were found to have an LOS that was 1.255 times shorter than the LOS of patients whose costs were reimbursed under the FFS method.
3. Patients whose costs were reimbursed under the casemix method were found to be 1.219 times less likely to be female than patients whose costs were reimbursed under the FFS method.

4. Patients whose costs were reimbursed under the casemix method were found to be 1.127 times younger than patients whose costs were reimbursed through the FFS method.

5. Patients whose costs were reimbursed using the casemix method were 4.630 times less likely to be surgical patients than patient whose costs were reimbursed under the FFS method.

6. Patients whose costs were reimbursed using the casemix method were 4 times less likely to be inpatients than patients whose costs were reimbursed using the FFS method.

7. Patients in the teaching hospital whose costs were reimbursed through casemix were 2.326 times less likely to have an unnecessary admission than patients whose costs were reimbursed through FFS.

The results of the multiple logistic regression analysis revealed that patients in the casemix group had lower hospital charges and shorter LOSs and were younger, less likely to be female, surgical patients, inpatients, and to have an unnecessary admission than patients in the FFS group.

## 4.3   Review of Billing Process

### 4.3.1 Review of Billing Costs

The researcher found many kinds of costs for the billing process in the data collected from the hospital financial report. The researcher divided those costs into 3 groups:

1. Human resources costs, which consisted of salaries, incentives, overtime fees, and the employee meal allowance. For the FFS method only, the cost of human resources also included fees and overtime fees for 3 officers from Public Health of Jakarta Province (PHOJP).

2. Transportation costs, which consisted of the costs associated with transportation for the billing officer to deliver the

hospital's claims to the payer's office. For the FFS method only, the transportation costs included the cost of renting cars to deliver the hospital's claim to the payer's office. For the casemix method only, the transportation costs included transportation costs for the verifiers.

3. Stationery costs, which consisted of the cost for copies, computer ink, stationery, and office equipment. For the FFS method only, the stationery costs included software maintenance and plastic wrap and containers for delivering claim documents to the payer's office.

The cost of human resources, transportation and stationery associated with the billing process are listed in table 4.28 for patients whose costs were reimbursed through the FFS method and in table 4.29 for patients whose costs were reimbursed through the casemix method.

Table 4.29 Cost of human resources, transportation and stationery in the billing process for patients whose costs were reimbursed under the FFS payment method

| No | Months | Human Resources | Transportation | Stationery |
|----|--------|-----------------|----------------|------------|
| 1. | January | 123,733,817.1 | 5,723,500.0 | 8,427,175.0 |
| 2. | February | 121,221,068.5 | 2,946,500.0 | 9,232,800.0 |
| 3. | March | 126,848,571.1 | 7,190,000.0 | 9,251,105.0 |
| 4. | April | 124,201,318.7 | 2,925,500.0 | 11,548,330.0 |
| 5. | May | 127,253,651.6 | 2,854,500.0 | 10,272,560.0 |
| 6. | June | 220,968,573.8 | 9,365,000.0 | 11,708,990.0 |
| 7. | July | 116,963,818.8 | 3,265,000.0 | 10,444,425.0 |
| 8. | August | 153,556,526.5 | 2,890,000.0 | 9,574,325.0 |
| 9. | September | 122,601,259.0 | 3,565,250.0 | 10,579,105.0 |
| 10. | October | 179,074,349.1 | 10,634,750.0 | 11,181,760.0 |
| 11 | November | 185,309,851.4 | 9,990,000.0 | 12,445,630.0 |
| 12 | December | 188,172,885.7 | 13,130,000.0 | 13,541,830.0 |
| | Total | 1,789,905,691.3 | 74,480,000.0 | 128,208,035.0 |

Sources: RSCM 2012. The Hospital Financial Report 2011

Table 4.30 Cost of human resources, transportation and stationery in the billing process for patients whose costs were reimbursed under the casemix payment method

| No | Months | Human resources | Transportation | Stationery |
|-----|-----------|-----------------|----------------|--------------|
| 1. | January | 49,850,030.0 | 3,125,000.0 | 353,350.0 |
| 2. | February | 51,145,629.2 | 3,125,000.0 | 428,340.0 |
| 3. | March | 50,689,025.7 | 3,125,000.0 | 341,045.0 |
| 4. | April | 49,362,716.5 | 3,125,000.0 | 497,560.0 |
| 5. | May | 50,645,629.4 | 3,125,000.0 | 415,120.0 |
| 6. | June | 51,904,235.0 | 3,125,000.0 | 519,580.0 |
| 7. | July | 60,456,495.3 | 3,125,000.0 | 386,830.0 |
| 8 | August | 54,145,298.4 | 3,125,000.0 | 405,235.0 |
| 9. | September | 54,928,840.2 | 3,125,000.0 | 578,775.0 |
| 10. | October | 54,279,654.9 | 3,125,000.0 | 812,375.0 |
| 11 | November | 59,828,241.3 | 2,750,000.0 | 1,002,500.0 |
| 12 | December | 80,708,629.2 | 2,875,000.0 | 970,440.0 |
| | Total | 667,944,425.0 | 36,875,000.0 | 6,711,150.0 |

Sources: RSCM 2012. The Hospital Financial Report 2011.

To obtain a better understanding of the billing process and its cost, this study compared the cost of human resources, transportation and stationery associated with the billing process for the FFS group and the casemix group in tables 4.29 and 4.30.

Table 4.31 Comparison of the cost of human resources, transportation and stationery in the billing process between patients whose costs were reimbursed under the FFS and casemix payment methods

| Cost | Mean or Median | Type of payment | | p |
|---|---|---|---|---|
| | | FFS (IDR) | Casemix (IDR) | |
| Human Resources | Median | 127,051,111 (Min–max 116,963,819– 220,968,574) | 55,662,036 (Min–max 49,362,717– 80,708,629) | 0.0001* |
| Transportation | Median | 4,644,375.0 (Min–Max 2,854,500– 13,130,000) | 3,125,000.0 (Min–max 2,750,000– 3,125,000) | 0.014* |
| Stationery | Mean | 10,684,002 (SD 1,478,250) | 559,262 (SD 236,787) | 0.0001** |
| Total cost of billing process | Median | 141,835,194 (Min–max 130,673,244- 242,042,564) | 56,612,174 (Min–max 52,985,277- 84,554,069) | 0.0001* |

* Mann-Whitney U test
**Two-tailed independent t-test

Significant differences were found between patients under the FFS method and patients under the casemix method for human resources costs in the billing process at p=0.0001. The median cost for human resources among billing administrators using the FFS method (IDR 127,051,111; min–max IDR 116,963,818.8– 220,968,574) was higher than the median human resources cost among billing administrators using the casemix method (IDR 55,662,036; min–max IDR 49,362,717–80,708,629). The median transportation cost in the billing process was higher under the FFS method (IDR 4,644,375; min–max IDR 2,854,500–13,130,000) than under the casemix method (IDR 3,125,000; min–max IDR 2,750,000–3,125,000) and significantly different at p=0.014. A significant difference was also found between the FFS method and the casemix method for stationery costs in the billing process at p=0.0001. The mean stationery cost in the billing process was higher under the FFS method (IDR 10,684,002; SD IDR 1,478,250) than under the casemix method (IDR 559,262; SD 236,787). The costs of human resources, transportation and stationery in the billing process were lower under the casemix method than under the FFS method. A significant difference was also found between the FFS method and the casemix method for the total cost of billing process at p=0.0001. The median total of billing process was higher under the FFS method (IDR 141,835,194; min-max IDR 130,673,244-242,042,564) than under the casemix method (IDR 56,612,174; min-max IDR 52,985,277-84,554,069).

The results described above comparing the cost of the billing process were combined with the results of the perception survey of billing administrators for a discussion of the billing process (sub-chapter 5.4.1). The perception survey of billing administrators were shown in the flow of billing process (table 4.36) which related to the cost of billing process.

To fulfil the study objectives, the costs for human resources, transportation, and stationery were aggregated into a total cost of billing per year. Then, the total cost of billing was divided by the total cost per case per year to reflect the cost of the billing process for one patient's bill under the FFS and casemix methods.

Table 4.32 Total cost of the billing process for patients' bill under the FFS and casemix payment methods

| No | Type of cost | Total cost of billing process per a year under FFS (IDR) | Total cost of billing process per a year under Casemix (IDR) |
|----|--------------|----------------------------------------------------------|--------------------------------------------------------------|
| 1 | Human Resources | 1,789,905,691 | 667,944,425 |
| 2 | Transportation | 74,480,000 | 36,875,000 |
| 3 | Copies, Computers and Software Maintenance | 128,208,035 | 6,711,150 |
| | Total | 1,992,593,726 | 711,530,575 |

Source. Financial Report 2011 (RSCM 2012).

There were 102,439 cases per year under FFS and 45,066 cases per year under casemix since 2011 (RSCM 2012). From the data above, the total cost of the billing process per year for patients whose costs were reimbursed by the FFS method was IDR 1,992,503,726 for 102,439 cases. The cost of one patient's bill under the FFS method was IDR 19,451. The total cost of the billing process per year for patients whose costs were reimbursed by the casemix method was IDR 711,530,575 for 45,066 cases. The total cost of one patient's bill under the casemix method was IDR 15,789.

To determine the impact of casemix implementation on the cost of billing in a teaching hospital, this study calculated the difference in the cost of billing between patients in the FFS group and patients in the casemix group:

$$\Delta \text{ cost of 1 patient's bill} = \text{cost of 1 patient's bill}_{FFS} - \text{cost of 1 patient's bill}_{casemix}$$
$$= \text{IDR } 19,451 - \text{IDR } 15,789$$
$$= \text{IDR } 3,662$$

$$\% \text{ cost of 1 patient's bill} = \frac{\Delta \text{ cost of 1 patient's bill} \times 100\%}{\text{cost of 1 patient's bill}_{casemix}}$$
$$= \frac{\text{IDR } 3,662.0 \times 100\%}{\text{IDR } 15,788.6}$$
$$= 23.2\%$$

The cost of one patient's bill under the FFS method was more expensive (IDR 3,662; 23.2%) than the cost of one patient's bill under the casemix method. In addition, the casemix method had a lower billing process cost and greater efficiency in hospital operational costs than the FFS method.

## 4.3.2 Review of Claims Reimbursed

All of the patients' bills were processed into the hospital's claims, which were delivered to the payers for verification and payment (see figures 2.1 and 2.6). The payers paid the hospital's claims based on the results of the verification process. Each payer had regulations for determining whether the hospital's claims would be approved or not.

The results of the study showing total hospital claims and paid claims are in appendix 11 and appendix 12 for inpatients and outpatients, respectively. Hospital claims and payments were aggregated into a percentage of total payments for 12 months for the FFS and casemix methods (Adams 2012).

$$\% \text{ of claims reimbursed} = \frac{\text{hospital claims paid by the payer}}{\text{hospital claims delivered by the hospital}} \times 100\%$$

The results of calculating the percentages of claims paid for 12 months under the FFS and casemix methods are shown in table 4.33. A result of 100% for percentage of claims paid indicates that all the hospital's claims were approved for payment by the payers.

Table 4.33 Percent of claims paid for outpatient and inpatient services
for patients under the FFS and casemix payment methods

| Month | Outpatient | | Inpatient | |
|---|---|---|---|---|
| | % Claim reimbursed by FFS | % Claim reimbursed by Casemix | % Claim reimbursed by FFS | % Claim reimbursed by Casemix |
| January | 98.9 | 100.0 | 97.2 | 100.0 |
| February | 99.6 | 100.0 | 91.5 | 100.0 |
| March | 99.3 | 100.0 | 95.8 | 100.0 |
| April | 99.2 | 99.9 | 90.8 | 100.0 |
| May | 99.1 | 99.9 | 89.8 | 100.0 |
| June | 97.8 | 99.9 | 91.5 | 100.0 |
| July | 96.7 | 100.0 | 92.6 | 100.0 |
| August | 96.6 | 100.0 | 87.1 | 100.0 |
| September | 96.5 | 100.0 | 84.9 | 100.0 |
| October | 89.8 | 100.0 | 87.9 | 100.0 |
| November | 98.3 | 100.0 | 97.9 | 100.0 |
| December | 99.4 | 100.0 | 91.6 | 100.0 |

To fulfil the study objective to compare the percentage of claims
paid between patients reimbursed under the casemix method and
the FFS method, this study compared the percentage of all claims
paid between the FFS method and the casemix method in 2011.

Table 4.34 Comparison of the percent of claims paid for patients under
the FFS and casemix payment methods in 2011

| Service | Type of Payment | | P |
|---|---|---|---|
| | % Claims Reimbursed Under FFS (N=102,439) | % Claims Reimbursed Under Casemix (N=45,066) | |
| Inpatient | 91.5 (87.1–97.2) | 100 | 0.0001* |
| Outpatient | 98.9 (89.8–99.6) | 100 (99.9–100) | 0.0001* |

* Mann-Whitney U test.

There were 102,439 hospital claims paid of patients whose costs were reimbursed under the FFS method with 3,883 claims of inpatient services and 98,556 claims of outpatient services. The hospital claims paid of patients whose costs were reimbursed under the casemix method were 45,066 claims which consisted of 4,387 claims of inpatient services and 40,679 claims of outpatient services. For outpatient services, the median percentage of claims paid was higher for patients under the casemix method (100%) than for patients under the FFS method (98.9%) (difference of 1.1%) and significantly different at p=0.0001. For inpatient services, the median percent of claims paid was higher for patients under the casemix method (100%) than for those under the FFS method (91.5%) (difference of 8.5%) and significantly different at p=0.0001. These results indicated that for both inpatient and outpatient services, casemix had a higher percent of claims paid than FFS.

### 4.3.3 Survey on Perceptions of The Billing Process

To fully describe the billing process in a teaching hospital, billing administrators were surveyed regarding their perceptions of the billing process. Of the respondents, 20 were billing administrators who were involved in billing under the FFS method, and 13 were billing administrators who were involved in billing under the casemix method. The respondents' profile is described in appendix 13. The scores for all respondents under the FFS and casemix methods are listed in appendix 14.

To examine the billing process, all scores were tested for normality, and median scores were calculated and then retranslated to the answers in the questionnaire. Those answers reflect the perceptions of the billing administrators regarding the billing process. The answers for the items in the questionnaire are listed in table 4.35.

Table 4.35 Billing administrators' perceptions of the patient billing process under the FFS and casemix payment methods

| No | Questions | FFS Method (N=20) | | Casemix Method (N=13) | |
|---|---|---|---|---|---|
| | | Median Scores | Answers | Median Scores | Answers |
| 1 | How many people on the billing staff are on your team? | 2.0 | 11 persons | 5.0 | 8 persons |
| 2 | The billing software used is..... | 4.0 | Easy to use | 5.0 | Very easy to use |
| 3 | The average number of patient billing documents processed in one day is.... | 1.0 | 250 documents | 1.0 | 250 documents |
| 4 | The average number of data items processed for one patient's bill is.... | 1.0 | More than 20 data items | 4.0 | 6 -10 data items |
| 5 | The summary report of the hospital's claims for one delivery is.... | 1.0 | More than 30 pages | 5.0 | Less than 15 pages |
| 6 | The hospital claim documents in one delivery to payers are.... | 2.0 | 5 large boxes (80x80x60 cm) | 5.0 | Less than 20 pages |
| 7 | The frequency of the hospital's claim delivery to payers in one month is.... | 1.0 | 5 times or more | 5.0 | Once |
| 8 | The payers'approval of a patients' billing documents when the patient discharged is as many as ..... | 1.0 | All patient billings | 5.0 | None |
| 9 | The length of time to prepare documents for one patient's bill is.... | 1.0 | 1 minute | 1.0 | 1 minute |
| 10 | The length of time to process documents in the billing software for one patient's bill is.... | 1.0 | 4 minutes | 4.0 | 1 minute |
| 11 | The length of time for the bill to be prepared and delivered to the payer (MOH/PHOJP) is...days after the service | 2.0 | 60 days | 4.0 | 30 days |
| 12 | Billing administrators receive the patient's bill from the inpatient service unit in...days | 4.0 | One month after patient discharged | 5.0 | One week after patient discharged |
| 13 | Billing administrators receive the verification result from the payer for the hospital's claim.... | 1.0 | More than 1 month after delivery | 3.0 | Two weeks after delivery |
| 14 | Billing administrators always receive the patient's bill with the medical chart | 1.0 | Strongly disagree | 4.0 | Strongly agree |
| 15 | Billing administrators always receive a fully completed medical chart | 2.0 | Disagree | 4.0 | Strongly agree |
| 16 | The billing process does not require a billing slip because billing is based on a diagnosis | 2.0 | Disagree | 4.0 | Strongly agree |
| 17 | Patients do not pay a contribution or a share of the bill's cost when they are discharged | 2.0 | Disagree | 4.0 | Strongly Agree |
| 18 | Does the billing administration process make it easy for patients? | 4.0 | Helpful | 4.0 | Helpful |
| 19 | Does the billing administration process make it easy for officers? | 4.0 | Helpful | 4.0 | Helpful |

To describe the steps of billing process, the data in table 4.35 are organized into the activities of the billing process in table 4.36. The perceptions of billing administrators are shown clearly on the activities of billing process for patients reimbursed under the FFS and casemix methods, and it was easier to use for discussion in chapter V

Table 4.36 Billing administrators' perceptions of the billing process activities under the FFS and casemix payment methods

| The activities of billing process | Questions | The billing administrators' perceptions under the FFS Method | The billing administrators' perceptions under the casemix method |
|---|---|---|---|
| Patient discharged | Administrators | 11 officers | 8 officers |
| | Software | Easy | Very easy |
| | No Contribution | Disagree | Agree |
| | Complete medical chart | Disagree | Strongly agree |
| | Administration for patients | Helpful | Helpful |
| Patient billing process for hospital claim | Patient documents received from wards | 1 month after patient discharged | 1 week after patient discharged continued......|
| | Receive medical chart with patient documents | Strongly disagree | Strongly agree |
| | No requirement for billing slips | Disagree | Strongly agree |
| | Patient billing documents sent in per day | 250 documents | 250 documents |
| | Data entry for one patient's bill | More than 20 data items | 6-10 data |
| | Time to prepare documents for one patient's bill | 1 minute | 1 minute |
| | Time to enter data for one patient's bill | 4 minutes | 1 minute |
| | Need approval from the payer | All patients' bills | None |
| | Administration for billing administrators | Helpful | Helpful |
| Claim and delivery | Summary of hospital's claim | More than 30 pages | Less than 15 pages |
| | Claim documents in one delivery to the payer | 5 large boxes (80x80x60cm) | Less than 20 pages |
| | Frequency of delivery for one month | 5 times or more | Once |
| | Time needed to deliver hospital's claim after patient discharged | 60 days | 30 days |
| Verification of payment | Time for payment verification | More than 1 month after delivery | Two weeks after delivery |

The survey questions were organized into five (5) dimensions, namely, tangibility, reliability, responsiveness, assurance, and empathy. A comparison was conducted between the billing administrators using the FFS method and those using the casemix method regarding their perceptions of the billing process.

Table 4.37 Comparison of perceptions of the billing process between billing administrators using the FFS and casemix payment methods

| Dimension | Type of payment | Median (min–max) | p |
|---|---|---|---|
| Tangibility | FFS | 3.5 (1–5) | 0.074 |
| | Casemix | 5.0 (2–5) | |
| Reliability | FFS | 1.0 (1–5) | 0.000* |
| | Casemix | 3.5 (1–5) | |
| Responsiveness | FFS | 1.0 (1–5) | 0.000* |
| | Casemix | 4.0 (1–5) | |
| Assurance | FFS | 3.0 (1–5) | 0.000* |
| | Casemix | 4.0 (2–5) | |
| Empathy | FFS | 4.0 (2–5) | 0.434 |
| | Casemix | 3.0 (2–5) | |

*Statistically significant $\alpha=0.05$; Mann-Whitney U test.

The comparisons in table 4.35 show that there were very significant differences between the perceptions of the FFS billing administrator group and the casemix billing administrator group with regard to the dimensions of reliability, responsiveness, and assurance at $p=0.0001$. However, there were no differences between the perceptions of the FFS billing administrator group and the casemix billing administrator group regarding the dimensions of tangibility ($p=0.074$) and empathy ($p=0.434$).

# V DISCUSSION

## 5.1 Introduction

Indonesia has several social insurance programmes that use different methods of payment. Two of the most common payment methods are fee-for-service (FFS) and casemix (WHO 2010). The FFS method is more widely known and has been used in Indonesia for a long time, while the casemix method was not known in Indonesia before the public health insurance (Jaminan Kesehatan Masyarakat or Jamkesmas) programme was launched in 2008. In 2013, the casemix method was designated as the official mechanism for hospital expense reimbursement within the platform of Indonesia's nationwide universal health coverage (UHC) programme, Jaminan Kesehatan Nasional (JKN or National Health Insurance) (MOH 2012).

FFS is the most popular payment method in the health service system. FFS is a retrospective payment method through which hospitals or other health providers are paid for every service they perform. The prices for all services rendered to a patient are calculated, and the total amount is then billed to the payer.

Hospital charges may vary between patients because each patient is treated individually according to his or her respective needs (PHOJP 2011, Adams 2012).

Unlike the FFS method, the casemix method applies a single charge to each episode of treatment in accordance with a clinical pathway. The casemix payment method consists of the costing and coding methods, which include the entire service cost that each patient has to pay (Adams 2012, MOH 2011). In Indonesia, the casemix method uses the charges listed in the Indonesian case-base groups (INA-CBGs) using the United Nations University (UNU)-Grouper software. The casemix method was established as the official mechanism for hospital charge reimbursement within the platform of National Health Insurance programme on January 1st 2014.

## 5.2 Review of Annual Hospital Reports

The costs of 22,643 outpatients and 3,883 inpatients were reimbursed through the FFS method, and the costs of 9,584 outpatients and 4,387 inpatients were reimbursed under the casemix method. The results show that most of the patients under the FFS method were female, with 11,438 female outpatients (50.5%) and 2,213 female inpatients (57.0%). Similarly, most of the patients under the casemix method were female, with 5,578 female outpatients (58.2%) and 3,096 female inpatients (70.6%). These results indicate that the patients whose costs were reimbursed under the FFS and casemix methods in 2011 were mostly female. This finding is due to the Jaminan Persalinan (Jampersal, maternity insurance) programme launched in May 2011 as a nationwide programme as part of the expansion of the Jamkesmas programme which already employed the casemix method (MOH 2011).

Based on the multiple regression analysis, patients in the casemix group were 1.219 times less likely to be female than patients in the FFS group. Even though the implementation of the maternity insurance programme using the casemix method began in May 2011, the FFS method was used for maternity insurance from January through April 2011. The review of the hospital's annual reports (table 4.2) revealed that under the FFS method, there were 11,438 female outpatients and 2,213 female inpatients, totalling 13,651 female patients. Meanwhile, under the casemix method, there were 5,578 female outpatients and 3,096 female inpatients, totalling 8,674 female patients.

In the FFS group, patients aged 0 to 4 years old (2,168 outpatients; 9.5% and 612 inpatients; 15.8%) and patients aged 45 to 49 years old (2,157 outpatients; 95%) represented the largest age groups. In the casemix group, patients aged 0 to 4 years old (1,018 inpatients; 23.1%) and patients aged 45 to 49 years old (925 outpatients; 9.7%) represented the largest age groups (table 4.1). The maternity insurance programme covers antepartum and postpartum services and the treatment of newly born babies, including immunizations (MOH 2011). These results indicate that patients aged 0 to 4 years old were associated with the maternity insurance programme. The national health policy, which launched the maternity health insurance programme in May 2011, influenced the national demographics of patients (WHO 2010).

The FFS payment method was used only for citizens of Jakarta province, and the highest numbers of referral patients were found in East Jakarta, with 6,846 outpatients (30.2%) and 1,267 inpatients (32.6%), and Central Jakarta, with 6,082 outpatients (26.9%) and 1,014 inpatients (26.1%) (table 4.4). These two regions of Jakarta are geographically close to the hospital that served as our study site, as the hospital is located in Central Jakarta and very near East Jakarta. The highest number of referral patients in the casemix group was found in West Java province with 1,582 inpatient cases (36.1%) and 5,858 outpatient cases (61.1%), which immediately borders Jakarta City (table 4.3). The provinces of West Java, Banten and Lampung directly border Jakarta Province—the location of the study site. Those three provinces represented the three highest referring areas for patients whose costs were reimbursed using the casemix method. From the data above, it appears that location is an important factor for accessibility in referring patients.

The multiple regression results indicated that the casemix method had 4.0 times fewer outpatients than the FFS method (table 4.28). The review of the hospital annual reports revealed that the total number of outpatients in the casemix group was 9,584 and that the total number of outpatients in the FFS group was 22,643. The FFS method was used for Jakarta citizens, who were located near the hospital that served as the study site. Meanwhile, the casemix system was used for citizens from areas outside the province of Jakarta. Thus, location was the main factor in access to the hospital; for Jakarta citizens, the close distance between their homes and the hospital made it easy for them to access the hospital services offered at the study site.

Outpatient diagnosis Z00-Z99.9 (factors influencing health status and contact with health services) was the most common diagnosis among patients in the FFS group (11,403 patients; 50.4%) and among patients in the casemix group (8,143 patients; 83.5%) (table 4.5). Meanwhile, the most common inpatient diagnoses for patients in the FFS group were C00-D48.7 (neoplasms) with 722 patients (18.6%); O00-O99.9 (pregnancy, childbirth, puerperium) with 580 patients (14.9%); and P00-P96.9 (certain conditions originating in the perinatal period) with 502 patients (12.9%) (table 4.7). The study site was the main teaching and national referral hospital, and this hospital has advanced medical equipment and specializes in oncology knowledge. The FFS payment method was used for Jakarta citizens in the Gakin (Keluarga Maskin, or poor families) programme. Thus, neoplasm cases were referred to the study site and represented the most common inpatient diagnosis among patients in the FFS group. The 2nd and 3rd most common diagnoses were O00-O99.9 and P00-P96.9, which were associated with maternity insurance cases that were covered under the Gakin programme in Jakarta until April 2011. At that time, those patients' diagnoses became part of the national maternity insurance programme under the Ministry of Health (MOH 2011).

The most common inpatient diagnoses among patients in the casemix group were O00-O99.9 (pregnancy, childbirth, puerperium) with 1,584 patients (36.1%) and P00-P96.9 (certain conditions originating in the perinatal period) with 764 patients (17.4%) (table 4.8). Both O00-O99.9 and P00-P96.9 represent the main diagnoses of the maternity insurance programme launched in May 2011. Thus, the high number of patients using the casemix method was mostly influenced by the enforcement of the national health policy (Mahendra & Trisnantoro, et al 2017).

The government's policy on health costs influences the demography of hospital patients (WHO 2010). The enforcement of social health insurance in Indonesia at the regional level and the national level, especially for poor citizens, truly helps patients to pay their hospital bills and encourages them to visit hospitals rather than clinics or nonmedical health providers. Table 2.2 shows that the number of hospital visits is increasing from year to year, i.e., 133,425,052 participants (51.8% of Indonesia's population) in 2014; 156,790,287 participants (60.8% of Indonesia's population) in 2015; and 171,930,254 participants (66.7% of Indonesia's population) in 2016. UHC, using the casemix method, has increased the availability of social health insurance in Indonesia (Mahendra & Trisnantoro, et al 2017, MOH 2017).

## 5.3    Review of Medical Services

### 5.3.1 The Impact of Medical Records

A medical record review was performed for the five most common diagnoses in order to fulfil one of the research objectives, namely, to determine and compare hospital charge and length of stay (LOS) for patients whose hospital bills were reimbursed using the casemix and FFS payment methods. The discussion of this sub-study covered the analysis of the five most common diagnoses for outpatient and inpatient services, the multiple logistic regression analysis and the survey on the perceptions of billing administrators. The researcher contends that the discussion should be very comprehensive and should include the results from the other sub-studies. A comprehensive discussion will result in a good conclusion for the medical review.

Of the five most common diagnoses for inpatient services, 3 were covered under the maternity insurance programme, namely, caesarean delivery (O.82.9), foetus and newborn affected by caesarean delivery (P03.4); and single spontaneous delivery (O80.9). Thus, maternity cases significantly influenced the demography of the patients. As noted earlier, the maternity insurance programme used the FFS method until April 2011 and changed to the casemix method in May 2011.

## a. The impact of hospital charges

Outpatient services usually consist of consultations, diagnostic support (laboratory services, X-rays, CT scans, MRIs, etc.), minor medical procedures, and pharmaceutical services (Hicks 2014). In table 4.10, the five most common diagnoses for outpatient services were Z09.8 (follow-up examination after other treatment for other conditions); Z08.9 (follow-up examination after unspecified treatment for malignant neoplasm); B24.0 (unspecified human immunodeficiency virus (HIV) disease); Z48.8 (other specified surgical follow-up care) and Z49.1 (extracorporeal dialysis). These outpatient services exhibited significantly different hospital charges for patients in the FFS group and patients in the casemix group (p=0.0001). All the median hospital charges for these five common diagnoses were higher for patients in the FFS group than for patients in the casemix group. Median hospital charge was higher for the FFS method than for the casemix method (table 4.11-4.15).

Also, hospital charges for inpatient services were significantly different between patient reimbursed by the FFS and casemix method in the five most common diagnoses (see table 4.16).

Median hospital charges were lower for patients under the casemix method than for patients under the FFS method (table 4.17-4.21).

Different payment types resulted in different hospital charges for reimbursement. The FFS method reimburses providers for delivering individual services (Beik 2015) and has been found to result in the prescription of more medicines per visit and higher costs in the public sector than in the private sector (Weissenberger and Thommen 2013).

The hospital in the study has implemented both type of payments for the National Drug Formulary (MOH 2010) and the prescription of generic drugs (MOH 2008) and for the Clinical Service Guidelines (RSCM 2011). However, different payment methods have different cost controls (Green 2017). Cost control determines how payment type decreases hospital costs and health expenditures for health care services.

Cost control by the payer or insurer is performed differently under the FFS method and the casemix method. To deeply examine cost control in this medical records review, the researcher combined the results of this sub-study with the results of the survey on the perceptions of billing administrators in table 4.35, namely, questions 8 and 17 and the "patient discharged" activities described in table 4.36.

The system of cost control by the payer was focused on not exceeding the maximum coverage amount (IDR 100,000,000) and was not able to optimally control the volume of prescribed medicine and the number of medical procedures. Cost control oriented towards a maximum coverage amount increasingly creates moral hazards. Overtreatment and overprescribing increase hospital 1 charges. The mechanism for hospital charge reform is one area of substantial efficiency that governments can address to deal with funding limitations (Yuki and Luca 2015).

Hospital charges under the casemix method consisted of all costs involved in one episode of patient treatment, including administration fees, doctor consultations, medical procedures, medical diagnoses, pharmacy care, medical wards, blood services, and other costs depending on the patient's diagnoses. An inpatient treatment episode started when the patient was admitted to the hospital and ended when the patient was discharged from the hospital (Berenson *et al* 2016). The charge was calculated after an episode of service or patient treatment was completed (Adams 2012). Unlike the FFS method, the casemix method implemented the single-episode charge approach to control costs per patient (Mathauer and Wittenbecher 2013).

Controlling the costs of medical services for patients under the casemix method has become the responsibility of hospitals as health providers, so cost control is mostly an internal affair within a hospital. Hospital officers do not know whether the payer will pay the hospital charge because the hospital charge can only be known at the end of each episode of patient treatment (Buck 2012). Implementing the single-episode hospital charge system produces more systematic cost control that begins with a patient's admission. Cost control is an integral part of each stage of service procedures, and this system helps increase awareness of cost control and promotes care in prescribing pharmaceutical supplies (medicines and medical equipment), establishing medical diagnoses (laboratory services, X-rays photographs, CT scans, MRIs), and planning medical procedures (Dewar 2017).

The single-episode charge is a good system for performing internal cost control within hospital management. Cost control is integral to the entire treatment process and is more economical because the payer does not need to provide or assign special officers for insurance approvals for cost control. Instead, hospital officers implement the single-episode charge system from the time of the patient's admission, and it has become the most common system using the casemix method. Casemix implementation has been found to control hospital costs (Stranges and Stocks 2008) and reduce financial risks through clinical pathways (Pirson, Martins *et al.* 2006). The casemix system also prevents over treatment, the use of too many procedures, and unnecessary procedures (Johri & Ng & Bermudez 2017), and it decreases overprescribing of pharmaceutical and generic drugs (Hopfe, Stucki *et al* 2016) and encourages cost containment (Buck 2012).

The discussion above also explains why the median hospital charges for the most five common diagnoses were higher under the FFS method than under the casemix method.

## b. The impact of length of stay

In table 4.16, the five most common diagnoses for inpatient services were O82.9 (caesarean delivery); P03.4 (foetus and newborn affected by caesarean delivery); Z51.1 (chemotherapy session for neoplasm); O80.9 (single spontaneous delivery) and C53.9 (malignant neoplasm of cervix uteri). Hospital charge and LOS for these diagnoses were significantly different for patients in the FFS group and the casemix group (p=0.0001). Median hospital charge and LOS were lower for patients under the casemix method than for patients under the FFS method (table 4.17-4.21). Thus, the different payment methods, i.e., FFS and casemix, resulted in different charges. In addition, a longer LOS increases hospital charges (Moreno-Serra & Wagstaff 2005).

For the FFS method, payers implemented cost control through the use of an essential services package (Paket Pelayanan Essensial or PPE), generic medicines, the National Drug Formulary, and the Hospital Formulary, through approval for expensive medicines and procedures, through the maximum benefit coverage of IDR 100,000,000, and through the verification of cost sharing when patients are discharged (PHOJP 2011). Due to the retrospective nature of the FFS method (Cashin 2015), hospitals as health providers calculate the total charge and continuously update it. For the FFS method, a patient or the patient's family must obtain payer approval since patients are admitted to the hospital until they are discharged, and an admission may include expensive procedures and treatments (PHOJP 2011).

According to the results of the survey on the perceptions of billing administrators, specifically question 8 in table 4.35 and the "patient discharged" activities in table 4.36, billing administrators using the FFS method perceived that all patient bills required payer approval. Approvals for procedures or drugs could have delayed treatment, resulted in a longer and inappropriate LOS and ultimately increased hospital charges under the FFS method.

When patients were discharged (see table 4.36), the payer also verified whether poor patients in outpatient and inpatient service units who had the Surat Keterangan Tidak Mampu (SKTM or recommendation letter for borderline poor people) letter were responsible for cost sharing (PHOJP 2011). Approval for cost sharing was obtained not through a computerized program but manually. The manual approval system required more time and had an impact by delaying patient discharge. This administrative procedure also inappropriately increased LOS under the FFS method, thus ultimately increasing hospital charges.

According to the discussion above, the FFS method increased LOS because of the many approvals needed from the payer. The results of the medical records review showed that the LOS for the five most common diagnoses was higher among patients whose costs were reimbursed by the FFS method than among patients whose costs were paid by the casemix method and that this difference was significantly different at $p=0.0001$. FFS correlates with an unnecessarily long LOS, and increasing LOS increases inefficiency in national health expenditures.

The results of study show that under the FFS method, payers were very dominant in cost control and controlled patient costs through many approvals. Consequently, hospital officials tended to delegate the role of cost control mostly to the payer. Thus, the role of an external party became greater than the role of the internal party with respect to cost control for patients under the FFS method. Even though the payer made its best effort to control costs, hospital charges and LOS were higher for patients under the FFS method than for patients under the casemix method. Moreover, cost control was not performed in a systematic way.

Many of the required approvals delayed medical services and prolonged LOS, which eventually increased the hospital charge.

FFS correlates with a pronounced increase in the volume of services and overall expenditures and unnecessarily long LOS (Amaro 2010), and this situation increasingly creates moral hazards in many countries and increases inefficiency in services (Murakami and Lorenzoni 2015). Overtreatment and overmedication are disadvantages of the FFS method, and they lead to high operational costs, inefficiency, and cost escalation (Campbell, Oona and Cegolon 2016).

Cost control under the case-mix method is performed differently than cost control under the FFS method. Based on the results of the survey on the perceptions of billing administrators, namely, question 8 in table 4.35 and the "patient discharged" activities in table 4.36, the billing administrators who used the casemix method reported that "No bills require approval". Approval for the casemix payment method was required only for severity level 3 cases, which must be verified by the hospital's medical committee and not by the payer (MOH 2011). The billing administrators who dealt with patients using the casemix method agreed with question 17 on the survey, "Patients do not pay a contribution or a share of the cost after discharge". The costs of patient treatment area burden not only for payers but also for patients. The FFS method increases inefficiency, which increases this burden on payers and patients (Berenson et al 2016). The answers reported above imply that patients did not need payer approval or verification regarding cost sharing for medical procedures or approval for discharge. The payer did not have a direct role in cost control for patients under the casemix method. Patients were discharged from the hospital without approval and without payments for cost sharing. These seamless administration procedures decreased LOS and prevented delays in treatment and in discharging patients, thus promoting lower hospital charges.

The casemix financing system is per episode, and the clinical pathway is the standard for services (Rozany & Yuliansyah &

Susilo 2017, MOH 2016). Implementing the casemix method with clinical pathways can control costs and reduce financial risks so that the use of medicines, pharmacy items, medical treatments, and cost containment efforts become more controllable (Mareno-Serra and Wagstaff 2005). Applying the casemix method with clinical pathways can also decrease unnecessary admissions, which has been proven to reduce health care costs (Richard and Pitluk 2008).

Systematic cost control in the casemix system, which is directly performed by the hospital, increases the speed of the medical care process because no approval is needed for patients to receive medical treatments, including when they are discharged. The casemix method reduces the number of days of hospitalization (Babic, Soldatovic, Vukovic *et al* 2015) and accelerates the turnover of hospital beds as part of bed management in a hospital (Duffield, Diers *et al*. 2009). The casemix system has also been shown to reduce average LOS (ALOS) by approximately 4% and bed-occupancy rate (BOR) by 5% (Moreno-Serra and Wagstaff 2005).

The discussion above describes the advantages of implementing casemix. The results of the study show that using the single-episode charge system with the casemix method led to seamless administration without the need for payer approval at each step of the medical care process. Cost control was also improved through internal hospital control. This system prevented delays in treatment and discharge, which decreased hospital charges and reduced LOS. Casemix implementation obviously benefits both patients and hospitals. Faster treatment helps to reduce the patient's medical costs (The NZ of MOH 2015), thereby decreasing inappropriate LOS (Wang & Stein & Hou *et al* 2017, Mossialos and Wenzl 2016, Amaro 2010).

The results of the multiple logistic regression analysis strengthened the results discussed above. The casemix method resulted in hospital charges that were 1.381 times lower than the hospital charges under the FFS method. The casemix method was also found to lead to an LOS that was 1.255 times lower than the LOS observed among patients whose charges were paid through the FFS method (table 4.28). Research has found that the FFS method has weaknesses in terms of controlling costs (Weissenberger 2013). The external control from insurers requires repeated approvals, including for discharging patients, which delays services and increases LOS. Even with these approvals, however, cost control under FFS is not optimal with regard to the use of medicines, examinations and medical treatments and LOS. The multiple regression analysis also revealed that the number of surgical patients under the casemix method was 4.6 times lower than the number of surgical patients under the FFS method. The FFS method can trigger overuse of patient services or overtreatment that can increase inefficiency in health financing (Carek & Bogan & Geesey 2008, Lenert 2010).

Based on the results of the medical record review and the discussion above, cost control is very important for reducing patients' medical costs. The internal single-episode charge system applied to patients under the casemix method was proven to be more effective in controlling patients' medical costs than the external cost control performed by payers for patients under the FFS method. This result shows that the FFS method has disadvantages, namely, the potential for uncontrolled treatment and inappropriately long LOSs. The study determined that casemix implementation promotes shorter LOSs and lower hospital charges compared to the FFS method. The single-episode charge system that was implemented as part of the casemix method improved cost control for health care services and became part of the hospital's internal control efforts.

## 5.3.2 The Impact of Unnecessary Admission

The discussion of unnecessary admission aimed to fulfil the research objective to compare the rates of unnecessary admission for patients whose costs were reimbursed using the casemix and FFS payment methods. In this study, unnecessary admission was defined as patients who were admitted to the hospital via the emergency room with an LOS of one day in the emergency room or in a third-class ward, were discharged from the hospital in better condition, were not referred to other health facilities, were not deceased, and had a diagnosis that was not included in the emergency diagnosis appendix in MOH Regulation Number 903/ MENKES/PER/V/2011 (MOH 2011).

The study results revealed that 357 patients under the FFS method had an LOS of 1 day during the year 2011, and of these, 257 (72.2%) were considered unnecessary admissions. For the casemix method, 407 patients had an LOS of 1 day, of whom 157 (38.6%) were considered unnecessary admissions (table 4.22). Unnecessarily admitted patients in both groups came from the same low-income group and used the same social health insurance benefit packages and public tertiary wards. For both payment methods in table 4.23, unnecessarily admitted patients were mostly female (FFS=166, 64.6%; casemix=124, 79.0%). The largest age cohort of patients was 40-50 years old, with 69 patients (26.9%) reimbursed through the FFS method and 55 patients (35.0%) reimbursed through the casemix method.

As a national referral hospital, the study site for this research is the highest referral hospital in Indonesia and accepts patients from lower-tier health facilities with referral letters. The referral system provides a means for lower-tier health facilities to refer patients to more advanced health facilities via referral letters. According to the Indonesia National Referral System (MOH 2011), true emergencies are necessary admissions, while unnecessary admissions are not true emergency cases. However, lower-tier hospitals that refer unnecessarily admitted patients to a higher-tier hospital increase hospital charges and health expenditures (Ham, Imison Jennings 2010; Babic, Soldatovic Vukovic et al 2015). Unnecessary admission is one health cost that contributes to inefficiency; moreover, hospital charges in a national referral hospital, such as the site investigated in this study, are more expensive than those in lower-tier health facilities. Patients admitted to a national-level hospital are therefore charged more than those admitted to a lower-level health facility (MOH 2016).

This study determined that referral letters from lower-tier health facilities were used by only 163 (63.4%) patients with an unnecessary admission whose charges were reimbursed under the FFS method. The remaining 94 (36.6%) unnecessary admissions were admitted directly to the emergency room without a referral letter. However, of the unnecessarily admitted patients whose costs were reimbursed under casemix, 155 (98.7%) patients had a referral letter from a lower-tier health facility, and only 2 (1.3%) patients were unnecessarily admitted without a referral letter (table 4.25). There were significant differences in the proportions of unnecessarily admitted patients admitted with and without referral letters between the FFS and casemix methods (p=0.0001). The rate of unnecessary admission without a referral letter was 28.2 times higher for the FFS system than for the casemix system (36.6%, 1.3%; p=0.0001).

The results of this study determined that the median hospital charge for patients under the FFS method was higher than that for patients under the casemix method, which led to higher costs for unnecessarily admitted patients under the FFS method than for those under the casemix method. Patients admitted to a national-level hospital are charged more than those admitted to a lower-level health facility (MOH 2016), and the FFS method increased hospital admissions by nearly 8%. Research has shown that a good referral system in one country decreased the cost of its national health care (Richard and Pitluk 2008).

A casemix system is defined as a system that reimburses per patient treatment episode; casemix systems are designed to create classes that are relatively homogenous with respect to resources used and that contain patients with similar clinical characteristics (Green 2016). The casemix method uses a single-episode charge approach, which begins when a patient is hospitalized and covers services until the patient is discharged from the hospital (Adam 2012). Single-episode charges include all medical treatments and procedures, diagnostic procedures, pharmaceutical services, consultations and hospital accommodations during the patient's stay in the hospital (Aljunid 2012). The hospital that provides care for the patient receives the full payment for one episode. However, hospitals that refer patients without a referral letter must pay for the medical treatment in the higher-tier referral hospital (MOH 2011). In addition, those patients' bills are not the payer's responsibility. Thus, the single-episode charge approach in casemix implementation increases adherence to the national referral system and decreases the rate of admissions without referral letters.

FFS is a retrospective reimbursement method in which providers (hospitals) are paid for each individual service they provide (Li, Lin & Masoudi et al 2015). Hospital charges vary among patients, as every patient receives care according to his or her individual needs (Aljunid 2012). Each individual service is insured by the payer without the single-episode consideration, so patients can receive medical treatment in multiple different health facilities. A hospital could refer a patient for only a certain medical treatment or diagnostic procedure (part of the patient's single-episode treatment) to a higher-tier referral hospital. FFS implementation favours unnecessary admissions. This study showed that among patients in the FFS group, 94 (36.6%) unnecessarily admitted patients were directly admitted to the emergency room without a referral letter. This study also revealed that the FFS method was 4.092 times more likely to be associated with unnecessary admission (table 4.22). This finding was strengthened by the results of the multiple logistic regression analysis, which indicated that the FFS method had a 1.87 times higher rate of unnecessary admission compared to the casemix method. The FFS method increased the admission of patients without referral letters and increased unnecessary admissions.

The results of this study also indicate that the median hospital charge for unnecessarily admitted patients under FFS (IDR 3,895,850) was higher than the median hospital charge for unnecessarily admitted patients under the casemix method

(IDR 3,600,514), and this result was significantly different at p=0.027 (table 4.24). The FFS method uses per procedure invoicing, which tends to lack cost controls and increases costs for patients (Campbell, Cegolon, Macleod, Benova 2016). FFS is also associated with increased service volume and overall cost as well as increased moral hazard in various countries (Medici and Murray 2010). Overtreatment and overmedication are drawbacks of the FFS method, and these disadvantages cause high operational costs, inefficiency and higher costs overall (Langenbrunner, Cashin, and O'Dougherty 2009).

The casemix method employs the single-episode charge approach with clinical pathways, which is a good system for implementing internal cost controls within hospital management to reduce patients' medical costs. The single-episode hospital charge approach in casemix implementation creates more systematic cost control and prevents overprescription, overtreatment, unnecessary procedures, and other unnecessary actions (Means 2016). Providers need to be more careful in managing costs, as the payer pays for each episode of patient treatment and not for each procedure. Casemix is associated with reduced hospital charges and reduced costs (Stranges and Stocks 2006). In this study, the casemix approach reduced unnecessary admissions and was associated with lower hospital charges.

The rate of unnecessary admission without a referral letters was 28.2 times higher for the FFS system than for the casemix system (36.6%, 1.3%; p=0.0001) (table 4.25). This result indicates that patients under the casemix method were referred to the hospital in stages from regional hospitals to provincial hospitals/ vertical hospitals to national central general hospitals—such as the study site—which are the highest referral hospitals in Indonesia. Unnecessary admission rates tended to be higher with the FFS method than with the casemix method; this was caused by the FFS referral system, which was not optimal and showed a tendency for patients in the surrounding community to come directly to the central national referral hospital without a referral letter. This led to an increase in health care cost inefficiency, as the national referral hospital has higher charges than primary health care facilities, regional hospitals, and provincial hospitals. Meanwhile, the referral system used with the casemix method was more aligned with the need for references at each stage, beginning with primary health care and continuing to national referral hospitals. Hospital charges for higher-level facilities are higher than those for lower-level health facilities, and referring patients with less complex cases to national-level referral hospitals can increase the health financing burden (Wibowo, 2013). Casemix implementation increased adherence to the referral system and the use of referral letters.

The results of this study revealed that implementing casemix with single-episode charges decreased the number of patients with an unnecessary admission and increased adherence to the national referral system compared to the FFS method.

## 5.4　Review of Billing Process

The review of billing consisted of 3 sub-studies, i.e., analyses of the cost of the billing process and hospital claims paid and a survey of the perceptions of billing administrators. The discussion combined these 3 sub-studies with the 3 related sub-studies described above in a comprehensive flowchart of the billing process to avoid repetition of the same subject.

### 5.4.1 The Impact of Cost of Billing Process

An analysis of the costs of billing was undertaken to fulfil the study objective to analyse the costs of the billing process under the casemix and FFS payment methods. In this study, costs were calculated from the billing receipts for every patient service processed by billing administrators until the hospital's claim was delivered to the payer. The billing administrators consisted of 2 separate groups, namely, billing administrators using the FFS method and those using the casemix method.

The costs of the billing process include the expenditures required to prepare patient bills until claim payment (RSCM 2011), and these costs are divided into direct costs and indirect costs. Direct costs are costs directly related to production activities in a unit, and their use can clearly be explored in a certain production unit. Indirect costs are costs indirectly related to service/production activities in a unit (Wenzel 2009). In this study, indirect costs were not included in the costs of billing based on the assumption that the indirect costs of the billing process were the same under the FFS and casemix methods. Some direct costs such as electricity, water, telephone, internet were also not included in the calculation of the costs of the billing process. This decision was made because these costs were jointly utilized in the billing process and because usage records were not available that separated the costs for the FFS and casemix method billing processes.

The results of study revealed 3 costs of the billing process for both the FFS and casemix methods, namely, costs for human resources, transportation and stationery. The human resources costs consisted of salaries, renumeration, and overtime fees as well as fees and overtime fees for verifiers under the FFS method. In table 4.31, the statistical analysis showed significant differences between patients whose costs were reimbursed via FFS and those whose costs were reimbursed via the casemix method in terms of human resources costs in the billing process at p=0.0001. The median human resources cost for billing administrators using the FFS method (IDR 127,051,111.4; min–max IDR 116,963,818.8–220,968,573.8) was higher than the median human resources cost for billing administrators using the casemix method (IDR 55,662,035.7; min–max IDR 49,362,716.5–80,708,629.2). According to the results for question 1 of the perception survey (table 4.35), there were 20 billing officers and 3 payer verifiers under the FFS method, while there were only 13 billing officers under the casemix method. The results for question 7 of the survey revealed that under the FFS method, the hospital's claims were delivered to payers 5 time or more per month, which increased the burden of the billing process. Moreover, this frequency resulted in a need for additional administrators or increased overtime hours and overtimes fees to deliver the hospital's claims. Thus, more billing administrators increased the human resources cost.

In addition, the responses to question 4 showed that for one bill under the FFS method, more than 20 data items had to be processed, while only 6-10 data items were processed for the casemix billing process. The FFS method required a billing slip, but the casemix method did not require a billing slip and was instead based on the diagnosis (question 16). The need for more data and documents resulted in more time managing each bill, thus increasing overtime fees in the billing process.

The billing process for the casemix method required the entry of 14 variables in a patient's bill including the patient's name, date of birth, age, and sex; type of treatment; date admitted to the hospital; date released from hospital; LOS; discharge status; the weight of babies aged 0–28 days (in grams);primary diagnosis; secondary diagnosis (if applicable); medical procedure; and code for special clinical major group (CMG) (if applicable). Of these 14 variables, 10 were obtained from the patient registration data, whereas only four variables (primary diagnosis, secondary diagnosis, medical procedure, and special procedure/drugs) were entered by the billing administrators into every patient bill. The total bills for all patients were aggregated and sent to the payer (MOH 2011, MOH 2016). The billing process for the casemix method does not require a service transaction receipt (table 4.36); instead, the total patient bill is determined from the coding results and the grouping of the patient data to generate the casemix charge (Buck, 2012; Green, 2016).

In question 10 of table 4.35, the billing process for the FFS method required 4 minutes to process data in the computer software, while the casemix method required only 1 minute to process data in the INA-CBG software. For the FFS method, the longer time required to process the data resulted in a need for more billing administrators and longer times for bill processing. This longer time for bill processing resulted in more work hours, which increased overtime hours and overtime fees. Thus, payment type influenced the billing process and the cost of the billing process. The FFS method had higher human resources costs than the casemix method.

Transportation costs consisted of costs associated with delivering the hospital's claims to the payer's office. The median transportation cost of the billing process was higher under the FFS method (IDR 4,644,375.0; min–max IDR 2,854,500.0–13,130,000.0) than under the casemix method IDR 3,125,000.0 (min–max IDR 2,750,000.0–3,125,000.0), and this result was significantly different at p=0.014 (table 4.31). For the FFS method, the responses to question 6 on the perception survey described the large number of documents included in one delivery to a payer, while the responses to question 7 revealed that claim deliveries were made 5 times or more per month, leading to the need for cars or rental cars for delivery (table 4.35). This greater frequency in claim delivery increased transportation costs. In contrast, hospital claims processed through the casemix method were delivered once per month and consisted of less than 20 pages. Cars were not needed to deliver the hospital's claim documents to the payer's office under casemix implementation, which reduced the operational costs of the billing process. Transportation costs for the billing process were higher under the FFS method than under the casemix method.

Stationery costs consisted of office equipment and copies and, for the FFS method only, the rental of containers and computer software. The statistical analysis showed a significant difference between the FFS and casemix methods for stationery costs in the billing process at p=0.0001. The mean stationery cost of the billing process under the FFS method (IDR 10,684,002.9; SD IDR 1,478,250.1) was higher than the mean stationery cost of the billing process under the casemix method (IDR 559,262.5; SD

236,787.0) (table 4.31). According to the results for question 5 on the perception survey of billing administrators (table 4.35), the FFS method required the preparation of more pagesof documents than the casemix method. The responses to question 6 revealed that under the FFS method, one delivery of the hospital's claim required 5 large boxes (80x80x60 cm) and plastic wrap; however, the casemix method did not require the delivery ofalarge number of documents to the payers. Thus, the billing process required more stationery and office equipment and was more complex under the FFS method than under the casemix method, resulting in a higher stationery cost for the billing process under the FFS method than under the casemix method.

The study results showed that the cost of the billing process per patient using the FFS method was IDR 19,451 and that the cost of the billing process per patient using the casemix method was IDR 15,789. The costs of the billing process under the casemix method were lower by IDR 3,662 (23.2%) than the costs of the billing process under the FFS method. Using the casemix method in the billing process increased efficiency in hospitals more than using the FFS method. The selection of payment method has an impact on cost reduction for services and on the costs of administration (Folland 2014).

Thus, the payment method influenced the cost of the billing process in the hospital. A simpler billing process expedites the process and reduces costs. The casemix system has effective and clear cost procedures and consistent incentives to achieve efficiency and leads to cost reductions (Buck 2012, Green 2016).

The discussion above proves the research hypothesis that the costs of the billing process are lower for patients under the casemix system of reimbursement than for patients under the FFS system of reimbursement. The costs of human resources, transportation and stationery in the cost of the billing process were lower under the casemix method than under the FFS method.

## 5.4.2 The Impact of Hospital Claims Reimbursed

This study compared the percentage of hospital claims paid between the FFS and casemix payment methods. Under the FFS method, all patient transactions were aggregated to generate a total patient bill, and all the total patient bills were then aggregated to create the hospital's claim, which was then sent to the payer (PHOJP2011, Green, 2016). The casemix method used medical charts with the INA-CBG Grouper software (MOH 2011) to send hospital claims to the payer.

A hospital's claims are delivered to a payer and are then verified and paid by the payer. The payer verifies the hospital bills and sends feedback regarding the verification results and the claims that will be paid (Buck 2012). The method of payment determines the amount of the claims paid by the insurer (Muharromah 2010) and may improve the efficiency of patient care, which will have an impact on lowering the medical costs borne by the insurer (Santoso 2016). Improving the speed and quality of the claim will influence hospital cash flow (Beik, 2013).

The results of the study showed that the median percent of hospital claims paid for inpatient services was higher for patients under casemix (100%) than for patients under FFS (91.5%) (a difference of 8.4%), and the difference was significant at p=0.0001. The median percent of hospital claims paid for outpatient services was higher under casemix (100%) than under FFS (98.9%) (a difference of 1.1%), and the difference was significant at p=0.0001(table 4.33). For the casemix method, if a patient's bill includes outpatient services and inpatient services on the same day, the charges for the outpatient services cannot be paid by the payer (MOH 2011 and 2016). This situation was described in the results of a study that found that hospital claims paid for outpatient services under the casemix method were 99.9% rather than 100%.

Verified hospital claims are then paid or rejected. For both the FFS and casemix methods, rejected claims could be sent back to the payer after the claims were completed or revised (MOH

2011, PHOJP 2011). The casemix method used the single-episode charge approach, which covered patients from the time they were admitted until they were discharged (Green 2016). This approach was discussed in the sub-study on the review of medical records.

The casemix method required the patient's medical chart for the billing process. Medical charts represent one of the documents that are the basis for coding all diagnoses and treatments and serve as a tool for determining the amount of hospital charges. According to the results for questions 14 and 15 on the perception survey of billing administrators (table 4.35), respondents using the casemix method agreed that they always received a completed medical chart, but the billing administrators using the FFS method had a different perception. Those respondents disagreed with the statement that they always received a complete medical chart. These perceptions indicate that the casemix method provided better medical records or charts than the FFS method because the medical records or charts were needed for the casemix billing system. The completeness and quality of medical record documents influence coding, grouping, and charges in the casemix method (Buck, 2012; MOH, 2016). Increasing the quality of medical record/medical chart writing is also one of the benefits of the casemix payment method used in hospitals (Aljunid, 2012; Buck, 2012).

Under the FFS method, the payer's approval officer in the hospital verified the hospital's claims, especially for expensive treatments, drugs/pharmaceutical supplies, diagnostics and medical procedures. The Gakin programme provided a maximum benefit of IDR 100,000,000. Unapproved health care treatments and those that exceeded the IDR 100,000,000 limit became the hospital's responsibility and were rejected by the payer (PHOJP 2011). The FFS method increased the overuse of services, but charges that exceeded the payer-insured maximum limitation became the patient's responsibility (Weissenberger, 2013). For these reasons, more hospital claims were delivered than paid under the FFS system: the percentage of hospital claims paid using the

FFS method was only 91.5% for inpatient services and 98.6% for outpatient services.

The different payment types had different regulations for billing and payment. The study results showed that the percentage of claims that were fully reimbursed were 8.5% higher for inpatients and 1.1% higher for outpatients under the casemix method compared to the FFS method. The payment method therefore has an impact on billing payments. The explanation above proves the hypothesis that the percent of claims paid was higher under the casemix method than under the FFS system.

### 5.4.3 The Impact of Billing Process

Of the billing administrators who responded to the survey on perceptions of the billing process, 20 were involved with billing under the FFS system, and 13 were involved with billing under the casemix method. The questionnaire consisted of 2 questions regarding tangibility, 6 questions about reliability, 5 questions on responsiveness, 3 questions regarding assurance and 3 questions about empathy. The results of the study showed no differences between the perceptions of billing administrators using the FFS method and those of the billing administrators using the casemix method regarding the tangibility (p=0.074) and empathy (0.434) dimensions (table 4.37). The results for the tangibility dimension revealed that even though the casemix method required fewer billing staff than the FFS method, the different types of billing software used for the two payment methods were easy to use. The results for the empathy dimension showed that the FFS and casemix methods made the billing process easy for patients and billing administrators.

In this discussion, the researcher focused more on the reliability, responsiveness and assurance dimensions, as significant differences were found between the perceptions of billing administrators under the FFS method and those of billing administrators under the casemix method regarding these dimensions (p=0.0001). When patients were discharged (table 4.36), those under the FFS method were responsible for a patient contribution, while patients under the casemix method did not have a patient contribution (question 17). The casemix method did not require approval of a contribution when patients were discharged. The casemix method also required complete medical charts as part of a patient's documents, while these were not available for the FFS method (questions 14 and 15). As discussed in the medical review, the casemix method was faster than the FFS method with regard to discharging patients. Casemix obviously benefits both patients and hospitals, and faster treatment helps reduce patients' medical costs (Busse *et al* 2013).

In the billing process, the average number of patient billing documents processed in one day was 250 documents for both the FFS and casemix methods (question 3). However, data processing for one patient's bill involved entering more than 20 data items, while the casemix method involved entering only 6-10 data items (question 4). In addition, the length of time to process one patient's bill in the computer billing software was 4 minutes for FFS and only 1 minute under the casemix method (question 10). The payment method selected has an impact on cost reduction for services and administration (Folland 2014). The casemix system has effective and clear cost procedures and consistent incentives to achieve efficiency and leads to cost reduction (Buck 2012, Green 2016).

Under the FFS method, the billing administrators received a patient's billing documents one month after the patient was discharged, but they received the billing documents one week after a patient was discharged under the casemix method (question 11). The FFS method required patients' billing slips, but the casemix method was based on the diagnoses in the medical chart and did not require patients' billing slips (question 16). For the FFS method, every transaction had a billing slip. The more services a patient received, the more billing slips were generated. Every service transaction was entered individually and consisted of the date, service unit, type of treatment, volume of activity, name of the doctor, hospital costs, hospital charges, and services (PHOJP 2011). By contrast, the casemix method required the medical chart for billing. The study found that the casemix method involved fewer documents to organize and enter into the billing software and required less time for the billing process. Thus, the casemix method makes the billing process easier by using the medical chart (Buck, 2012).

The FFS method involved managing more documents and delivering hospital claims more frequently than the casemix method, which increased the costs of the billing process since these activities increased the burden on and total work hours of employees. The number of billing administrators using the FFS method was higher than the number of the billing administrators using the casemix method. The high work load increased employee overtime costs under FFS. The higher number of employees and the increase in employees' overtime hours increased the human resources costs of the billing process for claims prepared using the FFS method.

In the claim delivery process (table 4.36), the summary of bills under the FFS method was more than 30 pages, which included as many as 5 large boxes of document appendices per delivery, and the frequency of bill delivery was as often as 5 times per month. By contrast, the patient bill summary under the casemix method was less than 15 pages with a document appendix that was fewer than 20 pages long, and the frequency of bill delivery was once per month (questions 5,6 and 7). The length of time to prepare and deliver a claim was 60 days under the FFS method, while it was only 30 days under the casemix method (question 11). The results of the perception survey showed that claim delivery under casemix reduced the number of documents and the frequency of claim delivery compared to FFS and that the process was faster under the casemix method than under the FFS method.

The verification time for the casemix method was 2 weeks, which was faster than the time of more than 1 month reported for the FFS method (question 13). The length of time required for the verification process depended on how many documents and data items had to be verified. For the FFS method, this process took more than one month due to the large number of documents, while the verification process took only 2 weeks for the casemix method, as it required fewer documents and less data. The payer verified the hospital's bills and sent feedback regarding the verified claims that would be paid (Buck 2012). The faster a hospital's claim is verified, the faster the hospital receives payment for the claim, which helps with the hospital's operational cash flow (Wendel, 2014). A faster billing process assists with hospital cash flow, and a delay in claim payments by a payer will disrupt a hospital's operational activities (Green 2013). The casemix method was associated with faster verification of the hospital's claims than the FFS method, which helped in maintaining the hospital's cash flow and operational activities.

The results described above reveal that the FFS method required processing every transaction for patient services through the payer's approval system, including cost sharing verification. Consequently, claim delivery preparation was longer (60 days), and the payer required more than one month to verify hospital bills due to the many documents included as attachments. However, under the casemix method, the billing process was simpler because it did not require approval from the payer. Patients' medical charts were sent to the billing administrators less than one week after the patients were discharged, and bill delivery preparation required 30 days. The payer needed only 2 weeks to provide feedback on the verification results for the hospital's claim. The payer payment process was easier and faster under the casemix method than under the FFS method because the casemix method involved fewer documents, and the process led to better cash flow for the hospital.

The discussion of the billing process above reveals that the FFS method was more complex and required more time than the casemix method. The casemix method was faster than the FFS method regarding patient discharge. The casemix method involved fewer documents to organize, less time for the billing process and fewer employees and overtime hours than the FFS method. Additionally, under the casemix method, claim delivery involved fewer documents, and claims were delivered less frequently. Moreover, the casemix method resulted in easier and faster verification of claims with fewer documents than the FFS method. These results prove the research hypothesis that claim processing for reimbursement is more complex under the FFS method than under the casemix system.

## 5.5 Compilation of Study Results

This discussion aims to fulfil the general study objective to examine the impact of implementing the casemix system for reimbursement of services in a teaching hospital in Indonesia. The researcher summarizes several sub-studies that were conducted to describe and compare the implementation of the casemix method to that of the FFS method for reimbursement of services in a teaching hospital.

Based on the research framework, there were two research area dimensions, namely, a review of medical records, consisting of 3 sub-studies (hospital charges, LOS, and unnecessary admissions), and a review of the billing process, consisting of 3 sub-studies (cost of the billing process, claims paid, and perception survey of the billing process). From the review of medical records, the researcher chose LOS and hospital charges as representative because both variables are health financing indicators (WHO 2010). Unnecessary admissions are associated with inpatient services and are therefore part of the LOS variable.

Based on the review of the cost of the billing process, the researcher contends that a relationship exists between the variable hospital claims paid and the variable hospital charge. The survey of the perceptions of billing administrators qualitatively described the billing process, which determined the cost of the billing process.

Therefore, the cost of the billing process was selected from the sub-chapter review on billing.

Finally, the researcher chose 3 variables, namely, LOS, hospital charge, and cost of the billing process for inclusion in a 3-dimensional figure called a "box-in-box" model. This box-in-box model consists of three axes: the "x" axis is LOS in days; the "y" axis is the hospital charge in IDR; and the "z" axis is the cost of billing in IDR. The following is the 3-dimensionalbox-in-box model:

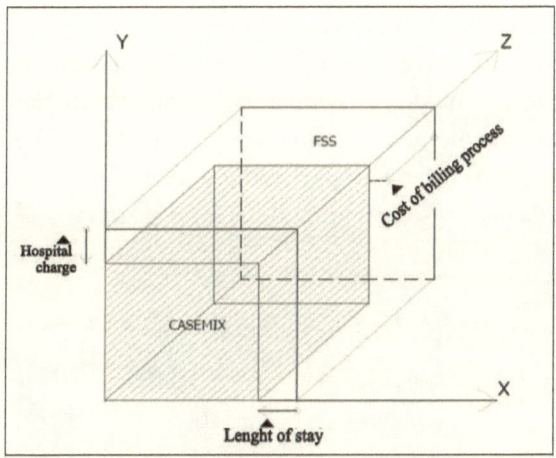

Figure 5.1 Box-in-box model of FFS and casemix
implementation in a teaching hospita

The box-in-box model describes the compilation of the results of the studies that were conducted to compare the implementation of the casemix and FFS methods. The LOS comparison results for the five most common diagnoses revealed that median LOS was longer under the FFS method than under the casemix method; this is shown on the "x" axis by the Δmedian LOS. The hospital charges for the five most common diagnoses were higher under the FFS method than under the casemix method; this is illustrated on the "y" axis by the Δmedian hospital charge. Finally, the costs of the billing process were IDR 3,662 higher under the FFS method than under the casemix method; this is shown on the "z" axis by the Δcost of the billing process for one patient bill.

Thus, in this model, the large box represents the FFS method, and inside this box is a smaller box that represents the casemix method. There are differences between the FFS and casemix method as shown by the Δmedian LOS from FFS to casemix, the median hospital charge from FFS to casemix, and the Δcost of the billing process for one patient bill (IDR 3,662) from FFS to casemix.

These results illustrate the efficiency of casemix implementation in a teaching hospital. The cost of the billing process can be improved as an efficiency indicator for payment method. With this box-in-box model, it is easier to describe the implementation of the casemix method for reimbursement in a teaching hospital, which leads to lower hospital charges, shorter LOSs and lower billing process costs compared to the FFS method.

# VI CONCLUSION AND RECOMMENDATIONS

In this chapter, the researcher concludes the discussion on the research results, hypothesis testing and research objectives. Moreover, recommendations are provided so that relevant parties, such as the Ministry of Health (MOH), hospital managers, clinicians and hospital workers, and researchers and academicians, can apply the research results. At the end of this chapter, the scope and the limitations of this research are explained.

## 6.1 Conclusion

Research was conducted on hospital charge reimbursement in a teaching hospital under two types of social health insurance using two different payment methods, namely, fee-for-service (FFS) and casemix. Both patient groups have the same benefit package, but their costs are reimbursed through different methods. To fulfil the research objectives, this study was divided into 2 sub-studies: a review of medical services (review of medical records and review of unnecessary admissions) and a review of billing (cost of billing, hospital claims paid and survey on perceptions of the billing process). This study proved all the proposed hypotheses and answered all the research questions.

### 6.1.1  Primary Objectives

The main objective of this study was to study the impact of implementing a casemix system for the reimbursement of services in a teaching hospital in Indonesia. This research was conducted with a comparative cross-sectional design between two (2) types of hospital charge reimbursement used for social health insurance. The results of comparisons between the FFS and casemix payment methods revealed differences in the impact of using the casemix method and the FFS method for charge reimbursement in a teaching hospital. The review of medical records and the review of billing found very significant differences between the implementation of the casemix approach and the FFS method in a teaching hospital.

The box-in-box model illustrates the impact of implementing the casemix method compared to the FFS method for charge reimbursement in a teaching hospital. With 3 main variables, length of stay (LOS), hospital charge and the cost of the billing process, the large box shows FFS, and the small box represents casemix. The difference in the sizes of the two boxes shows that implementing casemix in a teaching hospital leads to lower hospital charges, shorter LOSs and lower billing costs than implementing FFS.

### 6.1.2  Specific Objectives and Hypotheses

The demography of the samples was described using gender, age, referral area and primary diagnosis. For both the FFS and casemix methods, the number of female patients was higher than the number of male patients. For the FFS method, the largest proportion of patients were in the 0- to 4-year-old age range for both outpatient and inpatient services. For the casemix method, the largest proportion of inpatients were in the 0- to 4-year-old age group, and the largest proportion of outpatients were in the 45- to 49-year-old age group.

East Jakarta represented the most common referral area for patients under the FFS method, while West Java was the most common referral area for patients under the casemix method. The most common primary diagnosis for outpatient services was factors influencing health status and contact with health service (Z00-Z99.9) for both the FFS and casemix methods. Neoplasms was the most common primary diagnosis for inpatient services under the FFS method. Pregnancy, childbirth, puerperium was the most common primary diagnosis for inpatient services under the casemix method, and these services are related to the maternity insurance (Jaminan Persalinan, Jampersal) programme established in May 2011. The summary above fulfils the first specific study objective, namely, to describe the social demography and classification of primary diagnoses of patients whose costs were reimbursed using the casemix system under the social health insurance scheme.

## a. The impact of hospital charges and length of stay

The review of medical records for the five most common diagnoses in outpatient services revealed a very significant difference in hospital charges between patients under the FFS method and patients under the casemix method. All median hospital charges were higher for patients under the FFS method than for patients under the casemix method. In addition, for inpatient services, very significant differences were found between the FFS and casemix methods for LOS and hospital charge: hospital charge and median LOS were higher for patients under the FFS method than for those under the casemix method. This summary fulfils the second specific study objective to determine and compare hospital charges and LOS for patients whose charges were reimbursed through the casemix and FFS payment methods. This summary proves the first hypothesis—patients whose costs are reimbursed using the casemix method have shorter LOSs than those whose costs are reimbursed using the FFS method. This summary also proved the second hypothesis—hospital charges are higher under the FFS method than under the casemix payment method.

## b. The impact of unnecessary admission

The study on unnecessary admissions found a very significant difference between patients under the FFS method and patients under the casemix method regarding the proportion of unnecessary admissions. Patients in the casemix group were 4.1 times less likely to have an unnecessary admission than patients in the FFS group. The unnecessary admission rate was 1.87 times higher in the FFS group than in the casemix group (72.0%; 38.6%, p<0.001). The casemix method with single-episode charges increased adherence to the national referral system and the use of referral letters. The rate of unnecessary admission without a referral letter was 28.2 times higher for the FFS system than for the casemix system (36.6%, 1.3%; p=0.0001). Moreover, the casemix method promoted better adherence to the national referral system than the FFS method. Implementing the casemix method reduced unnecessary admissions and was associated with lower hospital charges. This summary fulfils the third specific study objective—to compare the rates of unnecessary admission for patients whose costs were reimbursed using the casemix and FFS payment methods. This summary also proves the third hypothesis, i.e., the unnecessary admission rate is higher for patients under the FFS method than for patients under the casemix method.

## c. The impact of billing

The costs of human resources, transportation, and stationery in the billing process were lower for patients under the casemix method than for patients under the FFS method. The costs of the billing process using the casemix method were lower by IDR 3,662 (23.2%) than the costs of the billing process using the FFS method. This explanation fulfils the fourth specific study objective, which was to analyse the cost of the billing process under the casemix and FFS payment methods, and proves the fourth hypothesis—that the cost of the billing process is lower for patients under the casemix reimbursement method than for patients under the FFS method.

The comparison of hospital claims paid for inpatient and outpatient services revealed a very significant difference between the FFS and casemix methods. The percentage of claims that were fully reimbursed was 8.5% higher for inpatients and 1.1% higher for outpatients under the casemix method compared to the FFS method. This explanation fulfils the fifth specific study objective, which was to compare the percentage of claims paid for patients whose costs were reimbursed under the casemix and FFS payment methods. The summary proves the fifth hypothesis—that the percentage of claims paid is higher under the casemix method than under the FFS method.

The survey of the perceptions of billing administrators found no difference between the two payment types regarding the tangibility and the empathy dimensions, but significant different were observed between the two payment types with respect to the reliability, responsiveness, and assurance dimensions. Compared to the casemix method, the FFS method resulted in slower patient discharge, more documents for bill processing, more time for bill processing, more approvals from the payer, more patient cost sharing, greater frequency in claim delivery, more documents for verification, and slower verification. These descriptions indicate that the billing process is more complex under the FFS method than under the casemix method. This discussion fulfils the sixth specific study objective, which was to compare the billing process for the casemix and FFS methods. This summary proves the sixth hypothesis that the billing process for reimbursement is more complex under the FFS method than under the casemix method.

## 6.2   Concluding Remarks

To make this research easy to understand, it was necessary to prepare a brief summary beginning with the background and ending with the recommendations based on the study results. This research was conducted in a main teaching hospital that used two (2) types of charge reimbursement for social health insurance through 2011. Beginning in 2012, the social health insurance programme has gradually transitioned to using the casemix approach, so 2011 was the last year that the two types of payment methods were used for the social health insurance system in Indonesia. For this reason, data from 2011 were used in the research.

In December 2013, the government of Indonesia designated the casemix payment method as the hospital charge reimbursement method for universal health coverage (UHC, a programme of the national health security system). The selection of the casemix method as the official payment method for UHC requires support from a study. Why was the casemix method selected? Is the casemix payment method better than the FFS payment method?

A comparative cross-sectional design was employed to compare the FFS payment method and the casemix payment method; the design included reviews of medical records for the five most common diagnoses for outpatient and inpatient services, unnecessary admissions, the cost of the billing process, and hospital claims paid and a survey of the perceptions of billing administrators.

Hospital charges for outpatient and inpatient services were lower under the casemix method than under the FFS method. In addition, LOS was lower under the casemix method than under the FFS method. The unnecessary admission rate was 1.87 times higher among patients under the FFS method than among patients under the casemix method (72.0%; 38.6%, p<0.001). The rate of unnecessary admission without a referral letter was 28.2 times higher for the FFS system than for the casemix system (36.6%, 1.3%; p=0.0001). The casemix method increased adherence to the national referral system, reduced unnecessary admissions and was associated with lower hospital charges.

The costs for human resources, transportation and stationery in the billing process were lower under the casemix method than under the FFS method. The cost of the billing process for one patient's bill was IDR 19,451 under the FFS method and IDR 15,789 under the casemix method. The cost of the billing process was IDR 3,662 (23.2%) lower under the casemix system than under the FFS system. The cost of the billing process correlated with the steps of the billing process, which was shown in the results of the survey on the perceptions of billing administrators.

The percentage of hospital claims paid for outpatient and inpatient services was higher under the casemix method than under the FFS method. The percentage of claims that were fully reimbursed was 8.5% higher for inpatients and 1.1% higher for outpatients under the casemix method than under the FFS method. The higher rate for claims paid increased the hospital's cash flow and the sustainability of hospital services.

The survey on billing administrators' perceptions of the billing process found no differences between the FFS method and the casemix method with respect to the tangibility and empathy dimensions, but significant differences between the two payment types were observed for the reliability, responsiveness, and assurance dimensions. Compared to the casemix method, the FFS method resulted in slower patient discharge, more documents for billing processing, more time for bill processing, more approvals from the payer, more patient cost sharing, greater frequency in claim delivery, more documents for verification, and slower verification. The FFS method had a more complex billing process than the casemix method with regard to patient discharge, the steps of the billing process, and claim delivery, verification of payment.

Based on the explanation above, the study results fulfil the main study objective and the specific study objectives as well as the 6 hypotheses of the research. This study also addressed the statement of the problem—that the casemix method for hospital charge reimbursement has more advantages than the FFS payment method as the official reimbursement method of the Indonesian UHC (Jaminan Kesehatan Nasional (JKN)) programme.

The study results show that the casemix method for hospital charge reimbursement has many benefits, namely, shorter LOSs, lower hospital charges, fewer unnecessary admissions, lower billing process costs, higher percentages of hospital claims paid, and less complexity in the billing process. The box-in-box model illustrating the compilation of results indicates that compared to the FFS method, the casemix method promotes lower hospital charges, shorter LOSs and lower billing process costs in a teaching hospital.

## 6.3  Limitations of The Study

The scope of this study was to examine the impact of implementing the casemix method for hospital reimbursement in a teaching hospital in Jakarta, Indonesia. A comparison of two types of payment—FFS and casemix—was conducted with data for two groups of patients using social health insurance in 2011, i.e., the Gakin (Keluarga Maskin, or poor families) and Jamkesmas (Jaminan Kesehatan Masyarakat) programmes. The study had the following limitations:

— The site study was only one teaching hospital, which did not represent all hospitals in Indonesia.
— The scope of the research included only low-income patients whose costs were reimbursed using the FFS

method or the casemix method in a main teaching and national referral hospital in 2011.

— The patients selected for the sample were outpatients during the period from January–March 2011 or inpatients during the period from January–December 2011.

— The patients selected for the research sample included only patients insured by a social health insurance programme. Patients whose costs were reimbursed through the casemix method were in the Jamkesmas programme, which included the maternity insurance and thalassemia insurance programmes, while patients whose costs were reimbursed through the FFS method were in the Gakin programme administered by Jakarta province.

— The data were obtained from the patients' documents or medical records, and the researcher did not observe the patients during the data collection.

— The number of samples in patients who were paid by the casemix payment method with ICD-10 code of B24 (Unspecified human immunodeficiency virus (HIV) disease) were only 38 samples. But the total number of samples in outpatients service of the five most common diagnoses among patients whose costs were reimbursed under the casemix payment method were 3,923 samples, and more than 675 samples as estimation sample size for the five most common diagnoses.

## 6.4 Recommendations

Since January 2014, Indonesia has offered UHC through a national health security programme, the JKN programme. Presidential Regulation Number 12 of 2013 states that the casemix payment method is the official method for charge reimbursement in the JKN programme. This research can offer insights and references for strategic policy making related to UHC in Indonesia. The research results can be considered in decision making, particularly with respect to the determination of charges and generally with regard to the development of UHC under the JKN programme in Indonesia.

The development of UHC through the national health security programme is intended to benefit all people in Indonesia. This goal requires strategic decision making at the national level (the government of Indonesia/the MOH), at the level of hospital management and among hospital employees and clinicians involved in the national health security programme. These study results support the academic research promoting the development of UHC.

Based on the results of this study, there are many recommendations for improving UHC and hospital management and for promoting the scientific development of provider payment methods through further studies.

## 1. The Ministry of Health of the Republic of Indonesia

These research results offer academic support that the selection of the casemix method for charge reimbursement for hospital services as stipulated by Presidential Regulation Number 12 of 2013 was correct. The research results indicate that the casemix method increases the efficiency of services, lowers billing costs and increases the percentage of claims paid. Cost control is an important consideration in maintaining the continuity of the UHC programme in Indonesia, and one of the strategic decisions for this programme is the selection of an appropriate payment method. The MOH determined that casemix is the appropriate payment method for hospital charge reimbursement for UHC in Indonesia.

It is useful to consider inflation and price increases when evaluating hospital charge reimbursement to ensure that hospital service quality remains high. This type of evaluation should become part of the annual agenda of the MOH and be included in the annual report of the health profile of Indonesia in the section on health financing.

The national referral system needs improvement so that teaching and national referral hospitals can be more beneficial for patients who truly need their services, even if those patients live far from the hospital. The regulations of the national referral system should be implemented with an integrated information technology system that includes family doctors, primary health care facilities, district hospitals, provincial hospitals, national referral hospitals and the central national referral hospital. To support the sustainability of Indonesian UHC, strategies are needed to transition curative care to promotive and preventive care, which are generally cheaper than curative care. Primary health care should systematically and continuously increase the role of promotive and preventive care. Decreasing curative care costs can increase efficiency in health care and improve health coverage to achieve UHC in Indonesia.

The cost of the billing process should become an indicator of efficiency in hospital management, especially in the UHC era. The cost of billing should be studied in greater depth to obtain more results on how billing is implemented in hospitals. Additionally, the results of this study should serve as a reference for the cost of the billing process under the FFS and casemix methods in hospitals.

Casemix is the official reimbursement method for the UHC programme; thus, it is necessary to continuously and systematically improve the understanding of managers, clinicians, and hospital employees regarding casemix as part of the national programme administered by the MOH. Such an effort would prove very useful to hospitals with respect to increasing knowledge about casemix and the implementation of the Indonesian case-base groups (INA-CBGs).

## 2. Hospital management

This research offers descriptions and knowledge for hospital managers regarding the implementation of two payment methods, FFS and casemix. Hospitals that are very familiar with the FFS method should gradually transition to the casemix method in the UHC era. Based on this research, managers should take appropriate strategic steps to manage hospitals and maintain service quality in the UHC era. Hospital management should develop good and efficient clinical pathways to manage patients and maintain quality, including controlling LOS and hospital costs.

Hospital management should also take strategic steps to evaluate the patient billing process in order to minimize operational costs and maintain the hospital's cashflow. The research results indicate that the cost of one patient's bill under the casemix method is approximately IDR 15,789; this result can become a basic indicator and can be adjusted for inflation. Similarly, the results of the survey on perceptions of the billing process can be used as descriptions and recommendations in the development of a billing process by hospital management.

Hospital managers should study the billing process used for the casemix method. A good understanding of the billing process can aid in maintaining a good cash flow and good quality of service. These research results should become references for the development of hospital management.

Cost control in hospitals should be improved by implementing single-episode charges using clinical pathways for medical services. An awareness of cost control and quality control should be built into the culture of the hospital.

## 3. Payers / insurers

The results of this study should serve as a reference to enrich the knowledge about casemix implementation in a teaching hospital. This study offers feedback for revising payer regulations for patients and hospitals. Medical services, the billing process, and payment verification should be performed faster and more seamlessly. Payer regulations should be evaluated and revised to promote less complex administration.

## 4. Clinicians

Clinicians should gain an understanding of the casemix system, as it is different from the FFS system that is very familiar to clinicians. The casemix method is based on single-episode treatments and requires clinical pathways. Clinicians should also develop good and rational clinical pathways. The implementation of clinical pathways helps clinicians determine appropriate patient services and procedures, aids in controlling treatment costs to reasonable and not excessive levels, and prevents overtreatment.

Doctors' awareness of the importance of writing complete and correct medical chart or records should be continuously promoted. In the casemix method, hospital charges are paid based on the diagnoses and procedures reported in the medical chart or record.

## 5. Hospital employees

Hospital employees' understanding of the casemix method should be improved. Changing from the FFS method to the casemix method requires different approaches to cost control. Hospital employees should use the results of this study to enrich the casemix method using single-episode charges and to improve cost control and the billing process. Hospital employees should also increase their awareness of quality and cost control.

Billing administrators should improve the technical billing process. The hospital's revenue depends on payments from the payer, and a good billing process supports the hospital's financial cash flow and maintains hospital services and activities.

## 6. Researchers and academicians

These research results can be used as a reference for scientific development and additional studies. However, future research should be conducted in non-teaching hospitals and private hospitals. All hospitals, including private and non-teaching hospitals, are involved in providing care in the UHC era.

This study examines an experience in one country that may rarely occur at another time or in other countries. The results of this study offer academic knowledge to enrich the understanding of casemix and FFS implementation in a teaching hospital among researchers and academicians. There are other large challenges regarding other countries' experiences for researchers to explore and include in the academic literature to improve knowledge about provider payment methods. Although many studies related to UHC focus on the casemix payment method, researchers and academicians should also pay attention to other types of payment methods, such as the FFS method.

This study also examined the billing process and the cost of the billing process, which have rarely been studied in the research on payment methods. Most of the studies on casemix have focused on the medical area; thus, researchers should pay greater attention to the billing process and the cost of the billing process, as these factors offer more insight into the advantages of casemix implementation. Researchers are also challenged to conduct additional studies on unnecessary admissions.

Using the results of this study as references, researcher are challenged to improve the science on provider payment methods by conducting further studies in other teaching hospitals, non-teaching hospitals, government hospitals and private hospitals.

# References

Adams, Wanda L. 2012. *Coding and Reimbursement. A simplified Approach.* Fourth Edition. Elsevier. St. Louis. Missouri. USA.

Aljunid, Syed Muhamed, et al. 2012. Modul 1: Introduction to Case-mix. International Centre for Case-Mix and Clinical Coding (ITCC), Faculty of Medicine, Universiti Kebangsaan Malaysia. http://unuiigh-Casemixonline.org.

Aljunid, Syed Muhamed,. et al. *Sistem Casemix Untuk Pemula. Konsep dan Aplikasi Untuk Negara Berkembang (Penerapan di Indonesia).* ITCC-UKM, Edition 2, Jakarta. 2011.

Amaro, Merced. 2010. Detailing unnecessary admissions to hospitals. www.californiahealthline.org/articles/2011/1/3/californiareleasesdata

Amaro, Merced. 2010. Detailing unnecessary admissions to hospitals. www.californiahealthline.org/articles/2011/1/3/californiareleasesdata.

Anderson G, Ikegami N. 2011. How can Japan's DPC inpatient hospital payment system be strengthened? Lesson from the US Medicare Prospective System. *A Report of the CSIS Global Health Policy Center*, Washington, DC.

Aryani, Y Anni., Rahmawati, Puput. 2010. The Effects of Participation in the Development of Performance Measures on Managerial Performance with Fairness Perception as a Mediating Variable: (An Empirical Study of Hospital Industry in Central Java, Indonesia). *Journal of Business and Policy Research. December.*5(2): 197 – 216.

Babic U, Soldatovic I, Vukovic D, Milicevic MS, Stjepanovic M, Kojic D, Argirovic A, Vukovic V. 2015. Comparative analysis of the current payment system for hospital services in Serbia and projected payments under diagnostic related groups system in urology. *Vojnosanit Pregl* 2015;72(3):251-257.

Babic U, Soldatovic I, Vukovic D, Milicevic MS, Stjepanovic M, Kojic D, Argirovic A, Vukovic V. 2015. Comparative analysis of the current payment system for hospital services in Serbia and projected payments under diagnostic related groups system in urology. *Vojnosanit Pregl* 2015;72(3):251-257.

Beik, Janet. 2013. *Health Insurance Today, A practical Approach.* Elsevier, 4th Edition. St Louis. USA.

Berenson, RA., Upadhyay, DK., Delbanco, SF., Murray, R. 2016. *Payment Methods: How They Work.* Research report of Urban Institute-USA.

Berg, LM., Ehrenberg, A., Florin, J. et al. 2018. Significant changes in emergency department length of stay and case mix over eight years at a large Swedish University Hospital. *International Emergency Nursing.* 43:50-55. Elsevier. USA.

Boachie, MK. 2014. Healthcare Provider-Payment Mechanism: A review of Literature. *Journal of Behaviour Economics, Finance Entrepreneurship, Accounting and Transport.* 2(3): 41-46. USA.

Buck, Carol J.; 2012. *The International Classification Diseases ICD-9-CM* volume 1,2,& 3 for Hospitals. AMA. Elsevier, USA.

Buck, Carol J.; 2012. *The International Classification Diseases ICD-10-CM* volume 1,2,& 3 for Hospitals. AMA. Elsevier, USA.

Busse, R., Geissler, A., Aaviksoo, A., et al. 2013. Diagnosis related groups in Europe: moving towards transparency, efficiency, and quality in hospitals?. *British Medical Journal.* June: 1-7. London. Doi: 10.1136/bmj.f3197

Busse, Reinhard., Geissler, Alexander., Quentin, Wilm., Wiley, Miriam. 2011. *Diagnosis-Related Groups in Europe: Moving towards transparency, efficiency and quality in hospitals.* European Observatory on Health Systems and Policies Series. USA: McGraw Hill.

Campbell, Oona, M.R., Cegolon, Luca.,et al. 2016. Length of Stay After Childbirth in 92 Countries and Associated Factors in 30 Low-and Middle-Income Countries; Compilation of Reported Data and a Cross-Sectional Analysis from Nationally Representative Surveys. *PLOS Medicine* 2016. March 8. United Kingdom. 2016.

Carek, Peter J., Boggan, Holly., Geesey, Mark E. 2008. Inpatient Care in a Community Hospital: Comparing Length of Stay and Costs Among Teaching, Hospitalist, and Community Services. *Family Medicine.* 40(2):119-124. Medical University of South Carolina. USA.

Cashin, C. 2015. *Assesing Health Provider Payment Systems: A Practical Guide for Countries Moving Toward Universal Health Coverage.* World Health Organization - Joint Learning Network. Washington.

Coelho, Julio CU., Fernandes, Fabina Marques., et.al. 2010. Appendectomy. Comparative Study Between A Public and A Private Hospital. *Rev. Assoc. Med Bras* 2010; 56(5):522-527. Brazilia.

Dahlan, Sopiyudin. 2009. *Statistik untuk Kedokteran dan Kesehatan. Deskriptif, Bivariat, Multivariat Dilengkapi Aplikasi dengan Menggunakan SPSS*. Edisi ke-4. Jakarta: Salemba Medika. Indonesia.

Dewar, Diane M. 2017. *Essentials of Health Economics*. 2nd Edition. Jones&Barlett Learning, USA.

Duenas, Alejandra. 2013. Cost Minimization Analysis. [In] *Encyclopedia of Behavioral Medicine*. Page 516-517. New York: Springer. USA.

Duffield, Christine., Diers, Donna., Aisbett, Chriss & Roche, Michael, Churn. 2009. Patient Turnover and Case Mix. *Nursing Economic*. May-June 27(3):185-191.

Fetter R, Shin Y., Freeman J an Averill R. 1980. Casemix Definition by Diagnostic – Related Groups Medical Care 18: 1-53.

Finkler S, Jones C, Kovner C. 2013. *Financial Management for Nurse Managers and Executives*. Elsevier Saunders: St. Louis. USA.

Folland, Sherman., Goodman, Allen C., Stano, Miron. 2014. *The Economic Health and Heath Care*. Pearson, seventh edition. Boston. USA.

Gerstman, Burt, B. 2015. *Basic Biostatistics. Statistic for Public Health Practice*. Second Edition. John & Bartlett Learning. California. USA. ISBN 1-284-02546-2

Green, Michelle A., Rowell, Jo Ann C. 2016. *Understanding Health Insurance A Guide to Billing and Reimbursement.* Cengage Learning, 13th Edition. Boston. USA.

Ham, Chris., Imison, Candace., Jennings, Mark. 2010. *Avoiding hospital admission, Lesson from evidence and experience.* The King's Fund https://www.kingsfund.org.uk/avoidinghospitaladmission

Hicks, Lanis L. 2014. *Economic of Health and Medical Care.* Sixth Edition. Jones & Bartlett Learning. Columbia. USA.

Hopfe, Maren., Stucki, Gerold., Marshall, Ric., et al. 2016. Capturing patients' needs in casemix : a systematic literature review on the value adding functioning information in reimbursement systems. *BMC Health Services Research* (16): p1-17.

Hosmer, D.W. and Lemeshow, S. 1989. *Applied Logistic Regression.* John Wiley and Sons. USA.

Jamieson, Susan. 2004. Likert Scales: How to Use Them. *Medical Education.* Vol 38: 1217-1218. USA.

Johri, Mira., Ng, Edmond, S.W., Bermudez-Tamayo, Clara., et al. 2017. A cluster-randomized trial to reduce caesarean delivery rates in Quebec: cost-effectiveness analysis. *BMC Medicine* (15): 1-9.

Kim SJ, Kim SJ, Han KT, Park EC. 2017. Medical costs, Cesarean delivery rates, and length of stay in specialty hospitals vs. non-specialty hospitals in South Korea. *PLOS one* November 30: 11 p. https://doi.org/10.1371/journal.pone.0188612

Landrum, Hollis., Prybutok, Victor. et al. 2009. Measuring IS System Service Quality with SERVQUAL: Users'Perceptions of Relative Imporance of the Five

SERVPERF Dimensions. Informing Science: *The Internasional Journal of an Emerging Transdiscipline.* Vol12(page 17- 35). USA. www.inform.nu/Articles/Vol12/ISJv12p017-35Landrum232.pdf.

Langenbrunner J, Cashin C, O'Dougherty S. *Overview: What, how, and who: an introduction to provider payment systems.* 2009. In: Langenbrunner J, Cashin C, O'Dougherty S, editors. Design and implementing health care provider payment system: how–to manuals. Washington DC: The World Bank; p. 1-26.

Lenert, Leslie. 2010. Transforming health care through patient empowerment. *Information Knowledge Systems Management.* Vol 8(1-4): 159-175.

Li Q, Lin Z, Masoudi FA, Li J, Li X, Diaz SH, Nuti SV, Li L, Wang Q, Spertus JA, Hu FB, Krumholz HM, Jiang L. 2015. National trends in hospital length of stay for acute myocardial infarction in China. *BMC Cardiovascular Disorder.*15:9. http://www.biomedcentral.com/1471-2261/15/9.

Limwattananon, Supon., Tangcharoensathien, Viroj. 2010. *Fee-for-service Payment Model: The Thai Experience and Evidence.* International Health Policy Program. Bangkok.

Louis D. Taroni F, Melotti R et al. 2008 Increasing appropriateness of hospital admissions in Emilia-Romagna region in Italia. *Health Services Research.* Vol 34(1): 405-415.

Lwanga, S.K., Lemeshow, S.1991. *Sample Size Determination in Health Studies.* World Health Organization. Geneva.

Lyles A. and Palumbo F. B. (1999) The effect of managed care on prescription drug costs and benefits. *Pharmocoeconomics* 15(2):129-40.

Mahendradhata, Yogi., Trisnantoro, Laksono., Listyadewi, Shita., Soewondo, P., Marthias, T., Harimurti, P., Prawira, J. 2017. The Republic of Indonesia Health System Review. The Health Systems in Transition. Vol 7(1). World Health Organization. Regional Asia. India. ISBN 978-92-9022-516-4. http://who.int/iris/bitstream/10665/254716/1/9789290225164-eng.pdf?sequence=1

Mathauer, Inke., Wittenbecher, Friedrich. 2013. *Hospital payment systems based on diagnosis-related groups: experiences in low and middle-income countries.* Bull World Health Organ 91:746-756A. DOI: http://dx.doi.org/10.2471/BLT.12.115931.

Means, Tracy. 2016. Improving quality of care and reducing unnecessary hospital admissions: a literature review. *British Journal of Community Nursing.* 21(6): 287-291. London.

Medici, Andre., Murray, Robert. 2010. Hospital Performance and Health Quality Improvements in São Paulo (Brazil) and Maryland (USA). *En Breve*; 156-Jun 2010. World Bank.

Moreno-Serra, Rodrigo., Wagstaff, Adam. 2009. *System-Wide Impacts of Hospital Payment Reforms. Evidence from Central and Eastern Europe and Central Asia. Impact Evaluation* Series no. 32. Policy Research Working Paper. The World Bank. Development Research Group. Human Development and Public Services Team. Washington DC. USA.

Moshiri, Hossein., Aljunid, Syed Muhammad., Amin, Mohd Rahmah., Ahmed, Zafar. 2010. Impact of Implementation of the Case-mix System on Efficiency of a Teaching Hospital in Malaysia. *Global Journal of Health Science* 2010; 2(2), October: 91-96.

Mossialos, Elias., Wenzl, Martin. 2016. 2015 *International Profiles of Health Care Systems*. London School of Economics and Political Science. Commenwhealth Fubd Pub. London.

Muharromah, Oktaviana. (2010). *Perbandingan antara metode pembayaran INA- DRG dengan FFS terhadap efisiensi dan mutu layanan untuk kasus Sectio Caesaria di RSUD Kota Bandung*. Tesis. Program Studi Kajian Administrasi Rumah Sakit. Fakultas Kesehatan Masyarakat Universitas Indonesia. Jawa Barat. Indonesia.

Murakami, Yuki., Lorenzoni, Luca. 2015. *Assessing the impact of case-based payment. [In] Case-based payment systems for hospital funding in Asia: an investigation of current status and future directions*. Peter Leslie and Dale Huntington (editors). Comparative Countries Studies. Volume 1(2). OECD - WHO.

Nevola, Adrienne; Pace, Cole; Karim, Salcema A; Morris, Michael E. 2016. Revisiting 'The Determinants of Hospital Profitability' in Florida. *Journal of Health Care Finance*. www.HealthFinanceJournal.com

Notoatmojo, Soekijo. 2010. *Metodologi Penelitian Kesehatan*. Jakarta: PT. Rineka Cipta. Indonesia.

Palmer G and Reid B. 2001. Evaluation of the performance of the Diagnostic–Related Groups and similar case-mix system: methodological issues. *Health Services Management Research* 14 (2) : 71-81.

Pett, Marjorie A. 2016. *Nonparametric Statistics for Health Care Research. Statistics for Small Samples and Unusual Distributions*. Second Edition. SAGE Publications. Inc. Washington DC, USA.

Pirson, Magali., Martins, Dimitri., Jackson, Terry., Dramaix, Michael., Lecler, Pol. 2006. Prospective Casemix-base funding, analy sis and financial impact of cost out liers in all-patient refined diagnosis related groups in three Belgian general hospitals. *Europe Journal of Health Economic.* 7:55–65.

Quinn, K. 2015. The 8 basic payment methods in Health Care. *Ann Inter Med.* PubMed. Aug 18; 163(4):300-6. Doi 10.7326/M14-2784. PMID: 26259075.

Richard F 3rd., Pitluk H., Collier P., et al. 2008. Reducing unnecessary Medicare hospital admission for chest pain in Arizona and Florida. *Profesional Case Management*;13(2), Mar-Apr:74-84. USA.DOI :10 .1097 /01. PCAMA. 0000314177.01661. b3. PMID:18344829.https://www.ncbi.nlm.nih.gov.

Rozany, Farida., Yuliansyah, Navis., Susilo, Siti J. 2017. The Guidence of clinical practice and clinical pathway as efficiency cost solution on Hernia Inguinalis, Appendisitis, and Sectio Caesarea cases in the Islamic Gondanglegi Hospital. *Jurnal Medicoeticolegal dan Manajemen Rumah Sakit (JMMR)* 6(2):122-129 DOI: 10.18196/jmmr.6135. http://journal.umy.ac.id/index.php/mrs.

Santoso, Budi Iman. 2016. *Penerapan Tarif INA CBG'S Era Jaminan Kesehatan Nasional Pada Efisiensi Biaya Kasus Sectio Caesariadi RS Cipto Mangunkusumo.*, Tesis Program Pasca Sarjana., Fakultas Kedokteran Universitas Gajah Mada, Yogyakarta.

Scheller-Kreinsen, David, MPP; Quentin, Wilm, MD, MSc, HPPF; Busse, Reinhard, MD, MPH. 2011. DRG-Based Hospital Payment Systems and Technological Innovation in 12 European Countries. www.elsevier.com/locate/jval. *International Society for Pharmacoeconomics and*

*Outcomes Research (ISPOR).* Published by Elsevier Inc. doi: 10.1016/j.jval.2011.07.001.

Sherpard, D.S., Hodgkin, D., Anthony, Y.E. 2000. *Analysis of Hospital Cost : A Manual for Managers.* WHO. Geneva.

Stranges, Elizabeth MS., Stocks, Carol. 2010. *Potentially preventable hospitalizations for acute and chronic conditions, 2008.* Agency for Healthcare Research and Quality. The Healthcare Cost and Utilization Project. November 2010. http://www.hcupus.ahrq.gov/potentiallyprevenable hospitalizationforacuteandchronicconditions.

Sulku, Seher Nur .2011. The Impacts of Health Care Reforms on the Efficiency of The Turkish Public Hospitals: Provincial Markets. *Munich Personal RePEc Archive,* Paper No. 29756. http://mpra.ub.uni-muenchen.de/29756/[22 March 2011].

The Central Bureau of Statistics (BPS). 2007. *The Indonesian Demography Survey 2007.* Jakarta. Indonesia.

The Cipto Mangunkusumo Hospital (RSCM). 2011. *The Clinical guidelines of the Cipto Mangunkusumo hospital.* Jakarta. Indonesia.

The Cipto Mangunkusumo Hospital. 2012. *The Annual the Cipto Mangunkusumo Hospital 2011.* Jakarta. Indonesia.

The Cipto Mangunkusumo Hospital. 2017. *The Annual the Cipto Mangunkusumo Hospital 2016.* Jakarta. Indonesia.

The Health Insurance Company (PT. Askes). 2012. *The Guidelines of Askes Programme.* Jakarta. Indonesia.

The Health Insurance Company (PT. Askes). 2013. The Development of Health Insurance in Indonesia. *Berita Askes.* http://askes.wordpress.com/perkembangan-asuransi-kesehatan-di-Indonesia.

The House of Representatives of the Republic of Indonesia (DPR-RI). 2004. *Social Health Insurance System, Constitution number 40.* Jakarta. Indonesia.

The Indonesia Ministry of Health. 2014. *The Drugs Formularium of The Jaminan Kesehatan Masyarakat programme.* Jakarta.

The Indonesia Ministry of Health. 2016. *The Guidelines of Indonesian Case Base Groups (INA-CBG's) in Jamian Kesehatan Nasional Programme.* Jakarta.

The Indonesian Company for Insurance (Jasindo). 2012. *The History of Health Insurance in Indonesia.* Jakarta: Jasindo.

The Ministry of Health. 2007. *The Indonesian Diagnoses Related Groups (INA-DRG's) Tariff.* Jakarta. Indonesia.

The Ministry of Health. 2008. *The Minimal Services Standards in hospitals.* Jakarta-Indonesia.

The Ministry of Health. 2010. *The compulsory of the generic drugs usage in the government health service facilities.* Jakarta. Indonesia.

The Ministry of Health. 2010. *The Indonesian Case Base Groups (INA-CBG's) Tariff 2010.* Jakarta. Indonesia.

The Ministry of Health. 2011. *The Guidelines of Jaminan Kesehatan Masyarakat Programme 2011.* Jakarta. Indonesia.

The Ministry of Health. 2011. *The Technical Guidelines of The Maternity Insurance (Jaminan Persalinan).* Jakarta. Indonesia.

The Ministry of Health. 2011. *The Technical Guidelines of The Thalassemia Insurance (Jaminan Pelayanan Thalasemia).* Jakarta. Indonesia.

The Ministry of Health. 2014. *The Guidelines of Jaminan Kesehatan Nasional (JKN) Programme 2014.* Jakarta. Indonesia.

The Ministry of Health. 2014. *The Guidelines of Pharmacoeconomy Review.* Jakarta. Indonesia.

The Ministry of health of The New Zealand. 2015. *The New Zealand Casemix System: an overview.* The New Zealand Casemix Project Group. New Zealand. ISBN 978-0-947491-19-2.

The Ministry of Health. 2015. *The Pattern of National Hospital Tariff.* Jakarta. Indonesia.

The Ministry of Health. 2016. *Data and Information of the Indonesian Health Profile 2011.* Jakarta. Indonesia.www. depkes.go.id/.../profil-kesehatan-Indonesia/profil-kesehatan-Indonesia-2016.pdf.

The Ministry of Health. 2016. *The Guidelines of Jaminan Kesehatan Nasional (JKN) Programme 2016.* Jakarta. Indonesia.

The Ministry of Health. 2017. Data and Information of the Indonesian Health Profile 2016. Jakarta. Indonesia. www.depkes.go.id/.../profil-kesehatan Indonesia/profil-kesehatan-Indonesia-2016.pdf. (13 Maret 2018)

The Ministry of Health. 2017. *Data and Information of the Indonesian Health Profile 2016.* Jakarta. Indonesia.www. depkes.go.id/.../profil-kesehatan-Indonesia/profil-kesehatan-Indonesia-2016.pdf. (1 April 2018)

The Ministry of Health. 2018. *National Health Insurance (Jaminan Kesehatan Nasional).* Jakarta. Indonesia.

The National Social Security Council (DJSN). 2012. *Himpunan Peraturan Sistem Jaminan Social Nasional (SJSN) dan Kelembagaan Dewan Jaminan Sosial Nasional (DJSN).* Jakarta. Indonesia.

The Public Health of Jakarta Province. 2011. *The Technical Guidelines of The Social Health Security and Disaster System in Jakarta Province.* Jakarta. Indonesia.

The Public Health of Jakarta Province. 2012. *The Jakarta Health Card Programme.* Jakarta. Indonesia.

The Public Health Office of DKI Jakarta Province (PHOJP). 2009. *The Technical Guidelines of The Social Health Security and Disaster System in Jakarta Province.* Jakarta. Indonesia.

The Social Health Implementation Agency (BPJS). 2016. *The Technical Guidelines of Jaminan Kesehatan Nasional (JKN) Programme.* Jakarta. Indonesia.

Timbie, Justin, W., Bogart, Andy., Damberg, Cheryl. L., Elliot, Marc, N., Haas, Ann., Gaillot, Sarah. J., Goldstein, Elizabeth, H., Paddock, Susan. M. 2017. Medicare advantage and fee-for-service performance on clinical quality and patient experience measures: comparison from three large state. *Health Services Research* 52(6): part 1. Health Research and Educational Trust. DOI: 10.1111/1475-6773.12787.

Wadhwa, vikas. Duncan, Morven. 2018. Strategies to avoid unnecessary emergency admissions. *British Medical Journal.* 362: k3. DOI: 10.1136/bmj. k3105.

Walker, R.A., 2011. *Categorical Data Analysis for Behavorial Social Science.* New York: Routledge Taylor and Francis Group.

Wang, Xin., Stein, Heller., Hou, Lie., Zou, Liying., et al. 2017. Caesarean deliveries in China. *BMC Pregnancy & Childbirth.*17: p 1-9. DOI: 10.1186/s 12884-017-1233-8.

Weissenberger N, Thommen D, Schuetz P, et al. 2013. Head-to-head comparison of fee-for-service and diagnosis related groups in two tertiary referral hospitals in Switzerland:

an observational study. *Swiss Medical Wlky*. May 17;143; w13790. USA: PubMed. PMID 23740092 DOI:10.4414/smw.2013.13790.

Weissenberger N, Thommen D, Schuetz P, et al. 2013. Head-to-head comparison of fee-for-service and diagnosis related groups in two tertiary referral hospitals in Switzerland: an observational study. *Swiss Medical Wlky*. May 17; 143;w13790. USA: PubMed. PMID 23740092 DOI:10.4414/smw.2013.13790.

Wendel, Jeanne; Donohue, William O'; Serratt, Teresa D. 2014. *Understanding Health Economics, Managing Your Career in an Evolving Healthcare System*. CRC Press. NW, USA.

Wenzel, Helmut. 2009. *Effectiveness Efficiency and Equity. Management in Health Care Practice a Handbook for Teachers*, Researchers and Health Professionals. Module 1.6 http://biecoll.ub.unibielefeld.de/volltextc/2009/ 2106/ pdf/article1.6.pdf

Wibowo, Bambang dan Mardiati Nadjib (2013). *Analisis Efisiensi pada selisih klaim INA CBG dan Pendapatan Rumah Sakit di 4 Rumah Sakit Kelas A, Studi Kasus Persalinan Sectio Caesaria*. The Faculty of Public Health – The Indonesia University. West Java. Indonesia.

Widi, Kartiko Restu. 2010. *Asas Metodologi Penelitian*. Yogyakarta.

World Health Organization (WHO), 2010. The world health report: *health systems financing: the path to universal coverage*. Geneva, World Health Organization.

World Health Organization (WHO). 2010. The world Health Report. *Health Systems Financing: the Path to Universal Coverage*. Geneva: World Health Organization.

World Health Organization. *The International Clasification of Disease ICD-10*. 2008.

World Health Organization. *The International Clasification of Disease ICD-9 Clinical Modification*. 2008. (15 Januari 2016)

Yip, WCM, Hsiao W, et al. 2010. Realignment of incentives for health-care providers in China. *The Lancet*. 375(9720):1120-30.

Zhang J. 2010. The Impact of diagnostic-related group-based prospective payment experiment: the experience of Shanghai. *Applied Economics Letters*. 17(18):1797-803.

# Appendix 1

Distribution of gender and age of patients with ICD-10 code Z09.8 for outpatient services whose costs were reimbursed under the FFS and casemix payment methods

| Items | Fee-for-service (N=3,785) (n,%) | Casemix (N=1,840) (n,%) |
|---|---|---|
| Gender: | | |
| Male | 1,845 (49.0%) | 931 (50.6%) |
| Female | 1,940 (51.0%) | 909 (49.4%) |
| | | |
| Age (years): | | |
| 0–10 | 667 (17.6%) | 277 (15.1%) |
| 10–20 | 414 (10.9%) | 303 (16.5%) |
| 20–30 | 450 (11.9%) | 350 (19.0%) |
| 30–40 | 461 (12.2%) | 210 (11.4%) |
| 40–50 | 634 (16.8%) | 291 (15.8%) |
| 50–60 | 695 (18.4%) | 260 (14.1%) |
| 60–70 | 371 (9.8%) | 112 |
| More than 70 | 93 (2.4%) | (6.1%) |
| | | 37 (2.0%) |

ICD-10 code Z09.8: Follow-up examination after other treatment for other conditions

# Appendix 2

Distribution of gender and age of patients with ICD-10 code Z08.9 for outpatient services whose costs were reimbursed under the FFS and casemix payment methods

| Items | Fee-for-service (N=1,321) (n,%) | Casemix (N=1,787) (n,%) |
|---|---|---|
| Gender: | | |
| Male | 448 (33.9%) | 496 (27.8%) |
| Female | 873 (66.1%) | 1,291 (72.2%) |
| | | |
| Age (years): | | |
| 0–10 | 171 (12.9%) | 143 (8.0%) |
| 10–20 | 46 (3.5%) | 125 (7.0%) |
| 20–30 | 61 (4.6%) | 73 (4.0%) |
| 30–40 | 200 (15.1%) | 385 (21.6%) |
| 40–50 | 429 (3%) | 496 (27.8%) |
| 50–60 | 304 (23.0%) | 388 (21.7%) |
| 60–70 | 92 (7.0%) | 138 (7.7%) |
| More than 70 | 18 (1,4%) | 39 (2.2%) |

ICD-10 code Z08.9: Follow-up examination after unspecified treatment for malignant neoplasm.

# Appendix 3

Distribution of gender and age of patients with ICD-10 code B24 for outpatient services whose costs were reimbursed under the FFS and casemix payment methods

| Items | Fee-for-service (N=348) (n,%) | Casemix (N=38) (n,%) |
|---|---|---|
| Gender: | | |
| Male | 217 (62.4%) | 20 (52.6%) |
| Female | 131 (37.6%) | 18 (47.4%) |
| | | |
| Age (years): | | |
| 0–10 | - | 4 (10.5%) |
| 10–20 | 12 (3.5%) | |
| 20–30 | 48 (13.8%) | 15 (39.5%) |
| 30–40 | 65 (18.7%) | 13 (34.2%) |
| 40–50 | 81 (23.2%) | 6 (15.8%) |
| 50–60 | 68 (19.6%) | |
| 60–70 | 69 (19.8%) | |
| More than 70 | 5 (1.4%) | |

ICD-10 code B24: Unspecified human immunodeficiency virus (HIV) disease.

# Appendix 4

Distribution of gender and age of patients with ICD-10 code Z48.8 for outpatient services whose costs were reimbursed under the FFS and casemix payment methods

| Items | Fee-for-service (N=344) (n,%) | Casemix (N=119) (n,%) |
|---|---|---|
| Gender: | | |
| Male | 194 (56.4%) | 65 (54.6%) |
| Female | 150 (43.6%) | 54 (45.4%) |
| | | |
| Age (years): | | |
| 0–10 | | |
| 10–20 | 18 (5.2%) | 5 (4.2%) |
| 20–30 | 57 (16.6%) | 19 (16.0%) |
| 30–40 | 62 (18.0%) | 22 (18.5%) |
| 40–50 | 79 (23.0%) | 26 (21.8%) |
| 50–60 | 62 (18.0%) | 23 (19.3%) |
| 60–70 | 60 (17.5%) | 22 (18.5%) |
| More than 70 | 6 (1.7%) | 2 (1.7%) |

ICD-10 code Z48.8: Other specified surgical follow-up-care.

# Appendix 5

Distribution of gender and age of patients with ICD-10 code Z49.1 for outpatient services whose costs were reimbursed under the FFS and casemix payment methods

| Items | Fee-for-service (N=116) (n,%) | Casemix (N=139) (n,%) |
|---|---|---|
| Gender: | | |
| Male | 70 (60.3%) | 78 (56.1%) |
| Female | 46 (39.7%) | 61 (43.9%) |
| | | |
| Age (years): | | |
| 0–10 | | |
| 10–20 | 7 (6.0%) | 7 (5.0%) |
| 20–30 | 18 (15.5%) | 22 (15.8%) |
| 30–40 | 20 (17.2%) | 25 (18.0%) |
| 40–50 | 29 (25.0%) | 33 (23.7%) |
| 50–60 | 16 (13.8%) | 24 (17.3%) |
| 60–70 | 24 (20.7%) | 26 (18.7%) |
| More than 70 | 2 (1.8%) | 2 (1.5%) |

ICD-10 code Z49.1: Extracorporeal dialysis.

# Appendix 6

Distribution of age of patients with ICD-10 code O82.9 for inpatient services whose costs were reimbursed under the FFS and casemix payment methods

| Age (years) | Fee-for-service (N=248) (n,%) | Casemix (N=497) (n,%) |
|---|---|---|
| 17–20 | 8 (3.2%) | 47 (9.5%) |
| 21–25 | 52 (21.0%) | 102 (20.5%) |
| 26–30 | 74 (29.8%) | 134 (26.9%) |
| 31–35 | 52 (21.0%) | 130 (26.2%) |
| 36–40 | 48 (19.4%) | 74 (14.9%) |
| 41–45 | 12 (4.8%) | 10 (2.0%) |
| More than 45 | 2 (0.8%) | |

ICD-10 code O82.9: Caesarean delivery.

# Appendix 7

Distribution of gender and age of patients with ICD-10 code P03.4 for inpatient services whose costs were reimbursed under the FFS and casemix payment methods

| Items | Fee-for-service (N=219) (n,%) | Casemix (N=136) (n,%) |
|---|---|---|
| Gender: | | |
| Male | 76 (34.7%) | 39 (28.7%) |
| Female | 143 (65.3%) | 97 (71.3%) |
| | | |
| Age: | | |
| 1–7 days | 195 (89.0%) | 102 (75.0%) |
| 8–14 days | 20 (9.1%) | 29 (21.3%) |
| 15–21 days | 2 (0.9%) | 2 (1.5%) |
| 22–28 days | 1 (0.5%) | 2 (1.5%) |
| More than 4 weeks | 1 (0.5%) | 1 (0.7%) |

ICD-10 code P03.4: Foetus and newborn affected by caesarean delivery.

# Appendix 8

Distribution of gender and age of patients with ICD-10 code Z51.1 for inpatient services whose costs were reimbursed under the FFS and casemix payment methods

| Items | Fee-for-service (N=210) (n,%) | Casemix (N=358) (n,%) |
|---|---|---|
| Gender: | | |
| Male | 96(45.7%) | 168 (46.9%) |
| Female | 114 (54.3%) | 190 (53.1%) |
| | | |
| Age (years): | | |
| 0–10 | 38 (18.1%) | 99 (27.7%) |
| 10–20 | 19 (9.1%) | 35 (9.8%) |
| 20–30 | 19 (9.1%) | 21(5.9%) |
| 30–40 | 35 (16.6%) | 73 (20.4%) |
| 40–50 | 49 (23.3%) | 81 (22.6%) |
| 50–60 | 39 (18.6%) | 45 (12.5%) |
| 60–70 | 10 (4.8%) | 4 (1.1%) |
| More than 70 | 1 (0.4%) | |

ICD-10 code Z51.1: Chemotherapy session for neoplasm.

# Appendix 9

Distribution of age of patients with ICD-10 code O80.9 for inpatient services whose costs were reimbursed under the FFS and casemix payment methods

| Age (years) | Fee-for-service (N=192) (n,%) | Casemix (N=280) (n,%) |
|---|---|---|
| 17–20 | 26 (13.6%) | 45 (16.1%) |
| 21–25 | 45 (23.5%) | 76 (27.1%) |
| 26–30 | 41 (21.3%) | 70 (25.0%) |
| 31–35 | 35 (18.2%) | 52 (18.6%) |
| 36–40 | 38 (19.8%) | 26 (9.3%) |
| 41–45 | 7 (3.6%) | 11 (3.9%) |

ICD-10 code O80.9: Single spontaneous delivery.

# Appendix 10

Distribution of age of patients with ICD-10 code C53.9 for inpatient services whose costs were reimbursed under the FFS and casemix payment methods

| Items | Fee-for-service (N=115) (n,%) | Casemix (N=102) (n,%) |
|---|---|---|
| Age (years) | | |
| 20–30 | 8 (7.0%) | 13 (12.7%) |
| 30–40 | 32 (27.8%) | 20 (19.6%) |
| 40–50 | 37 (32.2%) | 27 (26.5%) |
| 50–60 | 25 (21.7%) | 40 (39.2%) |
| 60–70 | 13 (11.3%) | 2 (2.0%) |

ICD-10 code C53.9: Malignant neoplasm of cervix uteri.

# Appendix 11

Total hospital claims and payments and percent of claims paid for inpatients whose costs were reimbursed under the FFS and casemix payment methods in 2011

| Month | FFS | | | Casemix | | |
|---|---|---|---|---|---|---|
| | Total Bill | Payment | % | Total Bill | Payment | % |
| Jan | 4,661,965,019.0 | 4,533,133,813.0 | 97.2 | 1,659,866,532.2 | 1,659,866,532.2 | 100 |
| Feb | 4,318,647,993.0 | 3,952,992,325.0 | 91.5 | 2,287,216,879.0 | 2,287,216,879.0 | 100 |
| Mar | 6,745,992,638.0 | 6,463,017,529.0 | 95.8 | 1,772,332,012.4 | 1,772,332,012.4 | 100 |
| Apr | 6,211,522,177.0 | 5,637,433,140.0 | 90.8 | 2,321,969,081.2 | 2,321,969,081.2 | 100 |
| May | 5,115,746,665.0 | 4,593,273,938.0 | 89.8 | 2,664,240,849.7 | 2,664,240,849.7 | 100 |
| Jun | 5,653,267,687.0 | 5,171,553,629.0 | 91.5 | 2,457,651,596.2 | 2,457,651,596.2 | 100 |
| Jul | 5,062,160,939.0 | 4,688,427,238.0 | 92.6 | 4,312,674,498.5 | 4,312,674,498.5 | 100 |
| Aug | 4,711,701,793.0 | 4,102,494,939.0 | 87.1 | 4,233,661,608.6 | 4,233,661,608.6 | 100 |
| Sep | 5,729,738,418.0 | 4,865,994,585.0 | 84.9 | 3,638,960,521.1 | 3,638,960,521.1 | 100 |
| Oct | 6,623,781,011.0 | 5,821,370,598.0 | 87.9 | 5,148,231,587.9 | 5,148,231,587.9 | 100 |
| Nov | 4,296,339,755.0 | 4,204,538,531.0 | 97.9 | 2,914,875,890.5 | 2,914,875,890.5 | 100 |
| Dec | 4,795,290,337.0 | 4,391,569,222.0 | 91.6 | 2,213,031,399.4 | 2,213,031,399.4 | 100 |

# Appendix 12

Total hospital claims and payments and percent of claims paid for outpatients whose costs were reimbursed under the FFS and casemix payment methods in 2011

| Month | FFS | | | Casemix | | |
|---|---|---|---|---|---|---|
| | Total Claim | Payment | % | Total Bill | Payment | % |
| Jan | 3,776,850,533.0 | 3,736,882,386.6 | 98.9 | 2,779,734,232.5 | 2,779,734,232.5 | 100 |
| Feb | 3,510,375,705.0 | 3,497,558,635.5 | 99.6 | 2,225,254,406.2 | 2,225,254,406.2 | 100 |
| Mar | 4,528,283,266.0 | 4,494,836,401.9 | 99.3 | 2,698,343,266.1 | 2,698,343,266.1 | 100 |
| Apr | 4,089,552,582.0 | 4,054,847,177.7 | 99.2 | 2,421,399,818.4 | 2,419,872,623.4 | 99.9 |
| May | 4,322,635,115.0 | 4,284,405,016.3 | 99.1 | 2,410,858,537.1 | 2,409,646,617.1 | 99.9 |
| Jun | 4,181,585,126.0 | 4,088,808,112.4 | 97.8 | 2,117,735,988.7 | 2,116,566,032.7 | 99.9 |
| Jul | 4,621,636,322.0 | 4,470,294,865.2 | 96.7 | 2,988,402,785.5 | 2,987,568,434.5 | 100 |
| Aug | 3,876,006,805.0 | 3,745,269,702.7 | 96.6 | 2,675,072,314.7 | 2,674,489,810.7 | 100 |
| Sep | 4,413,530,119.0 | 4,258,925,813.9 | 96.5 | 2,647,859,989.9 | 2,647,520,975.9 | 100 |
| Oct | 4,413,530,119.0 | 3,965,185,922.4 | 89.8 | 2,888,382,929.0 | 2,888,211,609.0 | 100 |
| Nov | 4,458,123,448.0 | 4,380,169,059.6 | 98.3 | 2,378,997,537.1 | 2,378,997,537.1 | 100 |
| Dec | 4,513,118,879.0 | 4,485,218,315.3 | 99.4 | 1,315,777,969.7 | 1,315,777,969.7 | 100 |

# Appendix 13

Profile of the perception survey respondents

| Profile | FFS (N=20) (n,%) | Casemix (N=13) (n,%) |
|---|---|---|
| Gender | | |
| Female | 9 (45%) | 5 (38.5%) |
| Male | 11 (55%) | 8 (61.5%) |
| | | |
| Age (years) | | |
| 20–30 | 10 (50%) | 11 (84.6%) |
| 31–40 | 4 (20%) | 2 (15.4%) |
| 41–50 | 4 (20%) | |
| 51 or more | 2 (10%) | |
| | | |
| Education | | |
| Up to Senior High School | 9 (45%) | 5 (38.5%) |
| Diploma | 5 (25%) | 6 (46.1%) |
| Post graduate | 6 (30%) | 2 (15.4%) |
| Length of Time as Billing Administrator (years) | | |
| 0–5 | 2 (10%) | 2 (15.4%) |
| 6–10 | 12 (60%) | 10 (76.9%) |
| 11–15 | 6 (30%) | 1 (7.7%) |

# Appendix 14

Scores for the survey on the perceptions of billing administrators under the FFS and casemix payment methods

**Q1 Tangibility: How many people on the billing staff are on your team?**

| Type of Payment | R1 | R2 | R3 | R4 | R5 | R6 | R7 | R8 | R9 | R10 | R11 | R12 | R13 | R14 | R15 | R16 | R17 | R18 | R19 | R20 |
|---|---|---|---|---|---|---|---|---|---|---|---|---|---|---|---|---|---|---|---|---|
| FFS | 1 | 1 | 1 | 1 | 5 | 5 | 5 | 5 | 5 | 5 | 2 | 2 | 2 | 2 | 1 | 1 | 3 | 1 | 5 | 5 |
| Casemix | 5 | 5 | 5 | 5 | 5 | 1 | 1 | 5 | 5 | 5 | 3 | 5 | 1 | | | | | | 5 | 5 |

**Q2 Tangibility: The billing software used is....**

| Type of Payment | R1 | R2 | R3 | R4 | R5 | R6 | R7 | R8 | R9 | R10 | R11 | R12 | R13 | R14 | R15 | R16 | R17 | R18 | R19 | R20 |
|---|---|---|---|---|---|---|---|---|---|---|---|---|---|---|---|---|---|---|---|---|
| FFS | 5 | 5 | 5 | 5 | 5 | 5 | 4 | 3 | 3 | 3 | 4 | 2 | 4 | 2 | 3 | 3 | 2 | 4 | 5 | 4 |
| Casemix | 5 | 2 | 2 | 5 | 5 | 5 | 5 | 5 | 5 | 5 | 2 | 4 | 4 | | | | | | | |

**Q3 Reliability: The average number of patient billing documents processed in one day is.....**

| Type of Payment | R1 | R2 | R3 | R4 | R5 | R6 | R7 | R8 | R9 | R10 | R11 | R12 | R13 | R14 | R15 | R16 | R17 | R18 | R19 | R20 |
|---|---|---|---|---|---|---|---|---|---|---|---|---|---|---|---|---|---|---|---|---|
| FFS | 1 | 1 | 1 | 1 | 1 | 1 | 1 | 1 | 1 | 1 | 2 | 2 | 2 | 2 | 1 | 1 | 1 | 1 | 1 | 3 |
| Casemix | 1 | 1 | 1 | 1 | 1 | 4 | 1 | 1 | 1 | 1 | 1 | 1 | 4 | | | | | | | |

## Q4 Reliability: The average number of data items processed for one patient's bill is ....

| Type of Payment | R1 | R2 | R3 | R4 | R5 | R6 | R7 | R8 | R9 | R10 | R11 | R12 | R13 | R14 | R15 | R16 | R17 | R18 | R19 | R20 |
|---|---|---|---|---|---|---|---|---|---|---|---|---|---|---|---|---|---|---|---|---|
| FFS | 5 | 1 | 5 | 5 | 5 | 5 | 5 | 5 | 5 | 5 | 5 | 5 | 5 | 5 | 5 | 5 | 5 | 5 | 5 | 5 |
| Casemix | 5 | 5 | 5 | 5 | 5 | 5 | 5 | 5 | 5 | 5 | 5 | 5 | 5 | | | | | | | |

## Q5 Reliability: The summary report of the hospital's claims for one delivery is....

| | R1 | R2 | R3 | R4 | R5 | R6 | R7 | R8 | R9 | R10 | R11 | R12 | R13 | R14 | R15 | R16 | R17 | R18 | R19 | R20 |
|---|---|---|---|---|---|---|---|---|---|---|---|---|---|---|---|---|---|---|---|---|
| FFS | 1 | 1 | 3 | 1 | 1 | 1 | 1 | 1 | 1 | 1 | 2 | 2 | 2 | 2 | 1 | 1 | 3 | 2 | 1 | 5 |
| Casemix | 1 | 1 | 1 | 1 | 1 | 1 | 1 | 1 | 1 | 1 | 1 | 1 | 1 | | | | | | | |

## Q6 Reliability: The hospital claim documents in one delivery to payers are....

| | R1 | R2 | R3 | R4 | R5 | R6 | R7 | R8 | R9 | R10 | R11 | R12 | R13 | R14 | R15 | R16 | R17 | R18 | R19 | R20 |
|---|---|---|---|---|---|---|---|---|---|---|---|---|---|---|---|---|---|---|---|---|
| FFS | 3 | 5 | 4 | 4 | 3 | 3 | 5 | 3 | 3 | 3 | 3 | 3 | 3 | 3 | 1 | 5 | 4 | 4 | 4 | 4 |
| Casemix | 3 | 3 | 3 | 3 | 3 | 4 | 1 | 3 | 3 | 3 | 4 | 5 | 1 | | | | | | | |

## Q7 Reliability: The frequency of the hospital's claim delivery to payers in one month is....

| | R1 | R2 | R3 | R4 | R5 | R6 | R7 | R8 | R9 | R10 | R11 | R12 | R13 | R14 | R15 | R16 | R17 | R18 | R19 | R20 |
|---|---|---|---|---|---|---|---|---|---|---|---|---|---|---|---|---|---|---|---|---|
| FFS | 1 | 1 | 1 | 1 | 1 | 1 | 1 | 1 | 1 | 1 | 1 | 1 | 1 | 1 | 1 | 1 | 1 | 1 | 1 | 1 |
| Casemix | 5 | 5 | 5 | 5 | 5 | 5 | 5 | 5 | 5 | 5 | 5 | 5 | 5 | | | | | | | |

## Q8 Reliability: The payers' approval of a patient's billing documents when the patient is discharged is as many as....

| | R1 | R2 | R3 | R4 | R5 | R6 | R7 | R8 | R9 | R10 | R11 | R12 | R13 | R14 | R15 | R16 | R17 | R18 | R19 | R20 |
|---|---|---|---|---|---|---|---|---|---|---|---|---|---|---|---|---|---|---|---|---|
| FFS | 3 | 3 | 1 | 1 | 1 | 1 | 1 | 1 | 1 | 1 | 1 | 1 | 1 | 1 | 1 | 1 | 1 | 1 | 1 | 1 |
| Casemix | 5 | 5 | 5 | 5 | 5 | 3 | 5 | 5 | 5 | 3 | 4 | 4 | 5 | | | | | | | |

## Q9 Responsiveness: The length of time to prepare one patient's bill is....

| Type of Payment | R1 | R2 | R3 | R4 | R5 | R6 | R7 | R8 | R9 | R10 | R11 | R12 | R13 | R14 | R15 | R16 | R17 | R18 | R19 | R20 |
|---|---|---|---|---|---|---|---|---|---|---|---|---|---|---|---|---|---|---|---|---|
| FFS | 1 | 1 | 1 | 1 | 1 | 1 | 1 | 1 | 1 | 1 | 1 | 5 | 1 | 1 | 5 | 5 | 1 | 1 | 1 | 3 |
| Cssemix | 1 | 1 | 1 | 1 | 1 | 4 | 2 | 1 | 1 | 1 | 1 | 5 | 5 | | | | | | | |

## Q10 Responsiveness: The length of time to process documents in the billing software for one patient's bill is....

| Type of Payment | R1 | R2 | R3 | R4 | R5 | R6 | R7 | R8 | R9 | R10 | R11 | R12 | R13 | R14 | R15 | R16 | R17 | R18 | R19 | R20 |
|---|---|---|---|---|---|---|---|---|---|---|---|---|---|---|---|---|---|---|---|---|
| FFS | 1 | 4 | 5 | 1 | 3 | 3 | 2 | 3 | 3 | 3 | 1 | 1 | 1 | 1 | 1 | 1 | 4 | 1 | 1 | 1 |
| Casemix | 4 | 4 | 4 | 4 | 4 | 5 | 1 | 4 | 4 | 4 | 2 | 4 | 1 | | | | | | | |

## Q11 Responsiveness: The length of time for the bill to be prepared and delivered to the payer (MOH/PHOJP) is...days after the service.

| Type of Payment | R1 | R2 | R3 | R4 | R5 | R6 | R7 | R8 | R9 | R10 | R11 | R12 | R13 | R14 | R15 | R16 | R17 | R18 | R19 | R20 |
|---|---|---|---|---|---|---|---|---|---|---|---|---|---|---|---|---|---|---|---|---|
| FFS | 5 | 2 | 1 | 1 | 1 | 1 | 1 | 1 | 1 | 1 | 1 | 1 | 1 | 1 | 5 | 5 | 5 | 1 | 5 | 5 |
| Casemix | 5 | 5 | 5 | 5 | 5 | 5 | 5 | 5 | 5 | 5 | 5 | 5 | 5 | | | | | | | |

## Q12 Responsiveness: Billing administrators receive the patient's bill from the inpatient service unit in...days.

| Type of Payment | R1 | R2 | R3 | R4 | R5 | R6 | R7 | R8 | R9 | R10 | R11 | R12 | R13 | R14 | R15 | R16 | R17 | R18 | R19 | R20 |
|---|---|---|---|---|---|---|---|---|---|---|---|---|---|---|---|---|---|---|---|---|
| FFS | 5 | 3 | 4 | 5 | 4 | 5 | 4 | 4 | 4 | 4 | 4 | 4 | 4 | 4 | 5 | 5 | 5 | 5 | 5 | 5 |
| Casemix | 5 | 5 | 5 | 5 | 5 | 5 | 5 | 5 | 5 | 5 | 5 | 5 | 5 | | | | | | | |

## Q13 Responsiveness: Billing administrators receive the verification result from the payer for the hospital's claim....

| Type of Payment | R1 | R2 | R3 | R4 | R5 | R6 | R7 | R8 | R9 | R10 | R11 | R12 | R13 | R14 | R15 | R16 | R17 | R18 | R19 | R20 |
|---|---|---|---|---|---|---|---|---|---|---|---|---|---|---|---|---|---|---|---|---|
| FFS | 1 | 1 | 1 | 1 | 1 | 1 | 1 | 1 | 1 | 1 | 1 | 1 | 1 | 1 | 1 | 1 | 1 | 1 | 1 | 5 |
| Casemix | 4 | 4 | 4 | 4 | 4 | 4 | 4 | 4 | 3 | 4 | 2 | 2 | 4 | | | | | | | |

## Q14 Assurance: Billing administrators always receive the patient's bill with the medical chart.

| Type of Payment | R1 | R2 | R3 | R4 | R5 | R6 | R7 | R8 | R9 | R10 | R11 | R12 | R13 | R14 | R15 | R16 | R17 | R18 | R19 | R20 |
|---|---|---|---|---|---|---|---|---|---|---|---|---|---|---|---|---|---|---|---|---|
| FFS | 4 | 1 | 2 | 4 | 1 | 1 | 1 | 1 | 1 | 1 | 1 | 1 | 1 | 1 | 2 | 1 | 1 | 1 | 1 | 1 |
| Casemix | 4 | 5 | 5 | 5 | 4 | 3 | 4 | 4 | 4 | 4 | 3 | 3 | 3 | | | | | | | |

## Q15 Assurance: Billing administrators always receive a fully completed medical chart.

| | R1 | R2 | R3 | R4 | R5 | R6 | R7 | R8 | R9 | R10 | R11 | R12 | R13 | R14 | R15 | R16 | R17 | R18 | R19 | R20 |
|---|---|---|---|---|---|---|---|---|---|---|---|---|---|---|---|---|---|---|---|---|
| FFS | 3 | 3 | 4 | 2 | 3 | 3 | 2 | 3 | 3 | 3 | 5 | 5 | 5 | 5 | 3 | 3 | 3 | 5 | 2 | 5 |
| Casemix | 4 | 5 | 5 | 5 | 4 | 3 | 4 | 4 | 4 | 4 | 3 | 3 | 3 | | | | | | | |

## Q16 Assurance: The billing process does not require a billing slip because billing is based on a diagnosis.

| | R1 | R2 | R3 | R4 | R5 | R6 | R7 | R8 | R9 | R10 | R11 | R12 | R13 | R14 | R15 | R16 | R17 | R18 | R19 | R20 |
|---|---|---|---|---|---|---|---|---|---|---|---|---|---|---|---|---|---|---|---|---|
| FFS | 4 | 3 | 5 | 4 | 4 | 4 | 4 | 4 | 4 | 4 | 3 | 3 | 3 | 3 | 3 | 3 | 5 | 5 | 5 | 5 |
| Casemix | 4 | 4 | 4 | 4 | 4 | 4 | 5 | 5 | 4 | 4 | 5 | 5 | 4 | | | | | | | |

## Q17 Empathy: Patients do not pay a contribution or a share of the bill's cost when they are discharged.

| | R1 | R2 | R3 | R4 | R5 | R6 | R7 | R8 | R9 | R10 | R11 | R12 | R13 | R14 | R15 | R16 | R17 | R18 | R19 | R20 |
|---|---|---|---|---|---|---|---|---|---|---|---|---|---|---|---|---|---|---|---|---|
| FFS | 5 | 5 | 5 | 5 | 5 | 5 | 4 | 3 | 3 | 3 | 4 | 2 | 4 | 2 | 3 | 3 | 2 | 4 | 5 | 4 |
| Casemix | 5 | 2 | 2 | 5 | 5 | 5 | 5 | 5 | 5 | 5 | 2 | 4 | 4 | | | | | | | |

## Q18 Empathy: Does the billing administration process make it easy for patients?

| | R1 | R2 | R3 | R4 | R5 | R6 | R7 | R8 | R9 | R10 | R11 | R12 | R13 | R14 | R15 | R16 | R17 | R18 | R19 | R20 |
|---|---|---|---|---|---|---|---|---|---|---|---|---|---|---|---|---|---|---|---|---|
| FFS | 4 | 3 | 5 | 3 | 3 | 3 | 4 | 3 | 3 | 3 | 4 | 4 | 4 | 4 | 2 | 3 | 4 | 4 | 3 | 5 |
| Casemix | 3 | 3 | 3 | 3 | 3 | 4 | 4 | 3 | 3 | 3 | 4 | 3 | 4 | | | | | | | |

| Q19 Empathy: Does the billing administration process make it easy for officers? | | | | | | | | | | | | | | | | | | | | |
|---|---|---|---|---|---|---|---|---|---|---|---|---|---|---|---|---|---|---|---|---|
| Type of Payment | R1 | R2 | R3 | R4 | R5 | R6 | R7 | R8 | R9 | R10 | R11 | R12 | R13 | R14 | R15 | R16 | R17 | R18 | R19 | R20 |
| FFS | 5 | 4 | 5 | 3 | 5 | 5 | 4 | 5 | 5 | 5 | 4 | 4 | 4 | 4 | 4 | 3 | 4 | 3 | 3 | 5 |
| Casemix | 3 | 3 | 5 | 5 | 3 | 3 | 4 | 3 | 3 | 3 | 4 | 3 | 4 | | | | | | | |

R= respondent

www.ingramcontent.com/pod-product-compliance
Lightning Source LLC
Chambersburg PA
CBHW030435290526
45786CB00001B/304